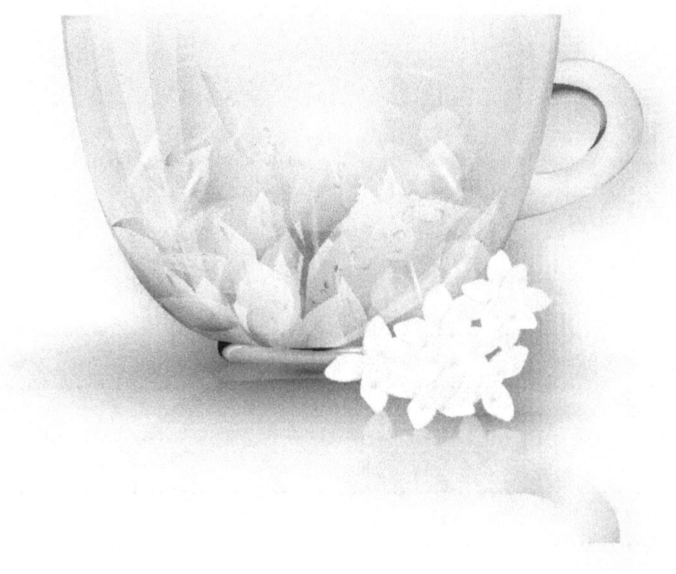

SPIRITED ALCHEMY OF TEA

The synergy of the western alchemical tradition and clinical herbalism leads to a truly holistic model of plant medicine. This is not a system focused on mere symptomatic treatment with herbs, but rather a comprehensive approach that equally works with the physical, energetic and spiritual elements of both people and plants. In this way, Alchemy takes your practice of herbalism to a deeper level where you are in fact supporting in the evolution of the soul.   "The School of Evolutionary Herbalism"

Author Cheri DeShaw

Herbal Teas for Health

Disclaimer

We hope you enjoy reading our reference book; however, we do suggest you read our disclaimer. All the material written in this report is provided for informational purposes only and is general in nature.

Every person is a unique individual and what has worked for some or even many may not work for you. Any information perceived as advice by must be considered considering your own set of circumstances.

The author or person sharing this information does not assume any responsibility for the accuracy or outcome of your use of the content.

Every attempt has been made to provide well researched and up to date content at the time of writing. Now all the legalities have been taken care of, please enjoy the content.

Results may vary. Information and statements made are for education purposes and are not intended to replace the advice of your doctor. If you have a severe medical condition or health concern, see your physician.

The research material has been from various sources on google and WebMD, they both seem to be reliable sources for up to date information.

For updated information please visit our websites.

Introduction

There is a chemistry and an **Alchemy to Tea**, discover yours Today.

I have always been a Tea drinker and over the past decades I have had an interesting life traveling to many different countries and experienced a variety of different Teas. Friends and family use to say why don't you just drink Coffee, I'd reply, Tea is so much healthier. Fifty years ago, the only Teas available if you dinned out in the USA were black teas. Now wherever you go there seems to be a wide variety and the popularity is growing. So, if you wish to indulge in Tea and would like to have a glimpse of what health properties are available in the different herbs, you will enjoy the information I have in the following pages. I have also included six different Spirited Alchemy Teas at the end of the book. If you wish to tract and create your own Tea formula's, start a journal on your Tea experience.

Enjoy and Drink Some Tea Today!

Herbal Teas for Health

The drink we know of as tea is a wholesome drink, and much better for us than most other hot beverages. However, as far as health benefits are concerned, herbal teas are a big step up again.

Herbal teas can be very refreshing, but beyond that that be viewed as medicine to treat conditions, or tonics to prevent them. Depending on the herbal infusion you choose, you can help relieve certain symptoms and ailments.

The secret is in knowing what type of herbal infusion or tea to take when you need to. For example, there are teas that stimulate and invigorate, and there are varieties that calm and relax.

This report discusses both types, as well as herbal teas that have been shown to be effective in helping reduce weight.

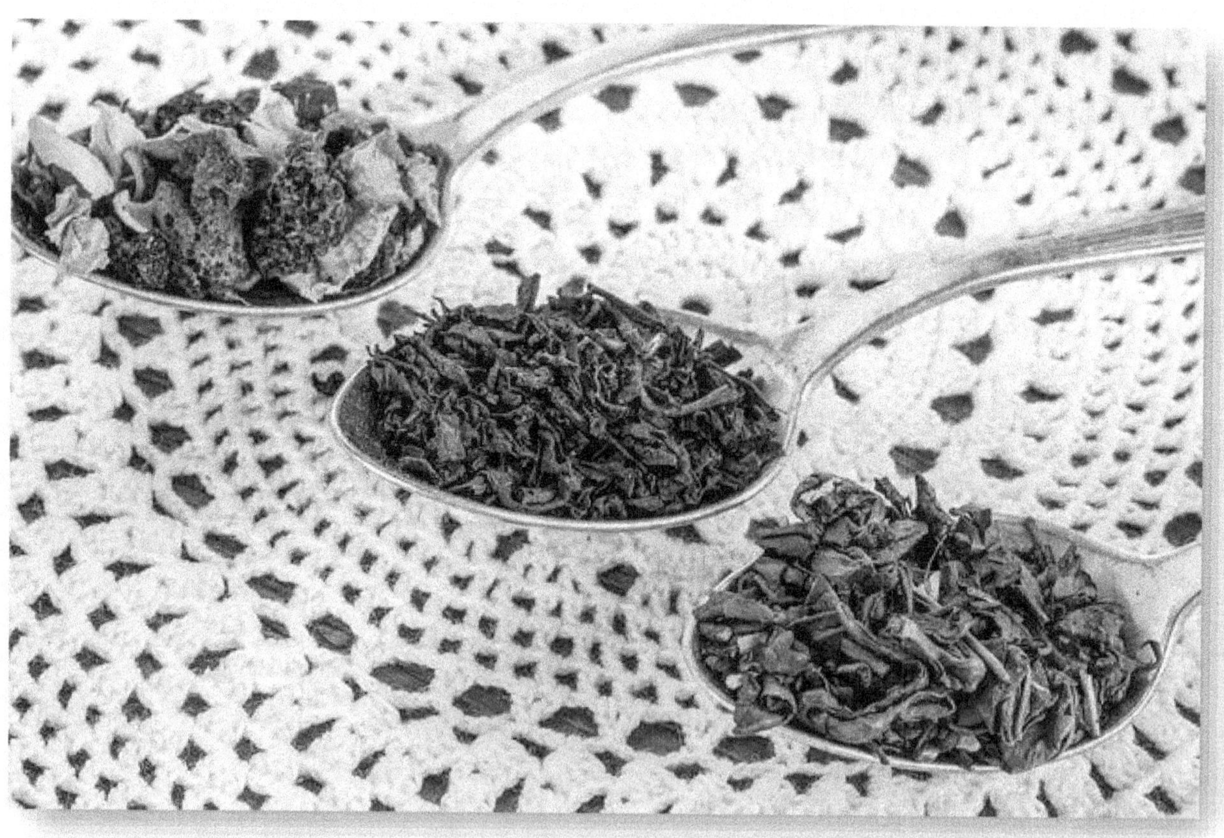

Herbal Teas for Weight Loss

Repeated studies, as well as masses of anecdotal evidence, show that certain herbal teas promote weight loss and boost the metabolism of the body. These teas not only help with weight loss, but they often provide the added benefit of lowering bad cholesterol levels and regulating blood sugar levels, while helping burn that excess body fat.

Drinking herbal teas for weight loss has many advantages compared to traditional slimming over-the-counter drugs and medications. They are a better alternative to try when wanting to lose weight and remain healthy!

Herbal teas can naturally assist with weight loss, but their added benefits far outperform the taking of weight loss pills. They can help keep the body and mind healthy and boost the immune system at the same time.

Some of the herbal teas that have effectively helped with weight loss are:

Siberian Ginseng Tea

Ginseng is an herbal tea famous for its actions in supporting the nervous system. However, this tea can also be placed into the weight loss tea group, as it helps to promote weight loss by balancing sugar levels and controlling appetite.

Ginger Tea

Ginger tea is also known for its ability to encourage weight loss. It detoxifies the body of excess toxins, neutralizes free radicals, cleanses the digestive system and kidneys, and improves blood circulation. Ginger possesses properties that increases metabolic rate to help burn calories that might otherwise become bodyfat.

Nettle Tea

This herbal tea is also rich in Vitamin C and antioxidants. Nettle tea induces weight loss by detoxifying the body and suppressing cravings and appetite.

Dandelion Tea

Dandelion is rich in antioxidants and vitamins and balances the body's pH levels.

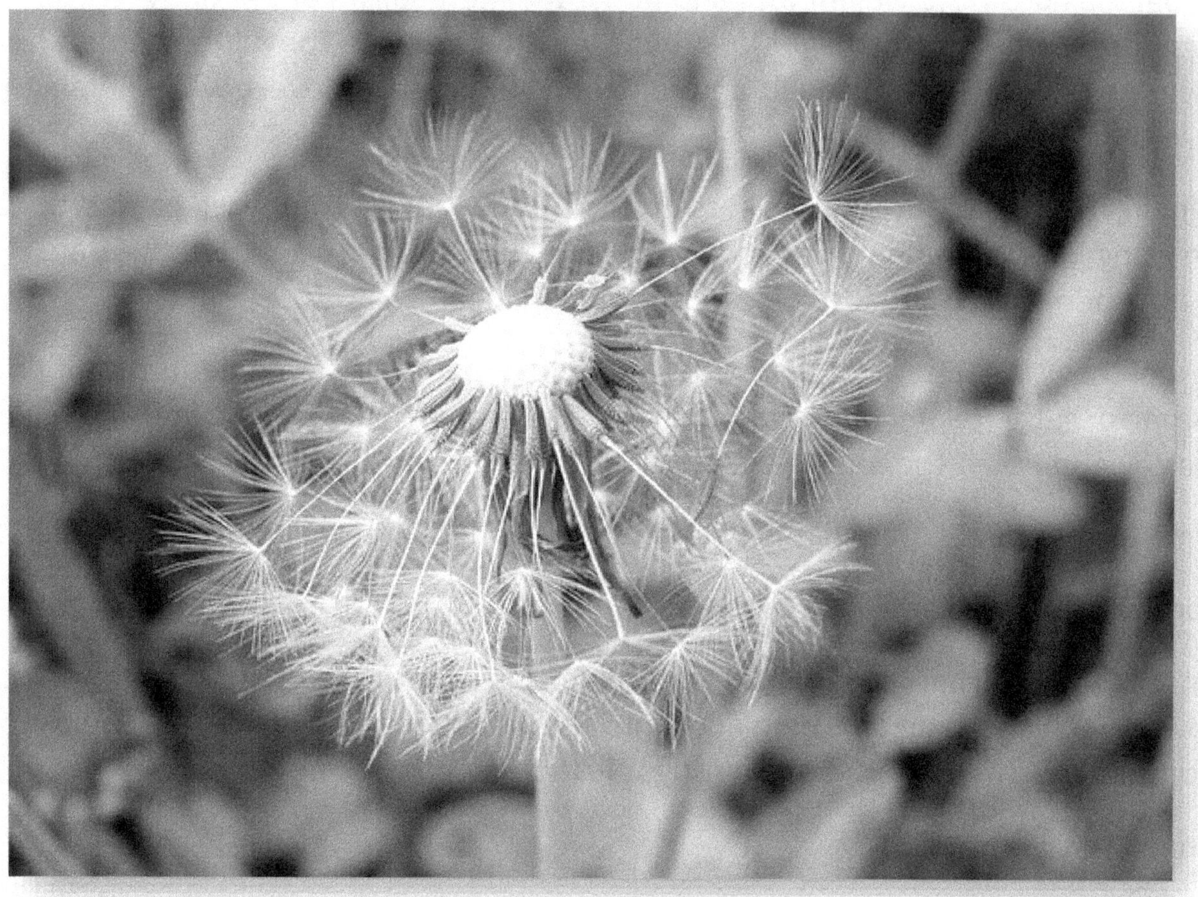

The acid balancing properties of dandelion tea aids in body detoxing and helps regulate bowel movements.

Fennel Seed Tea

Fennel seed tea is another soothing herbal tea that cleanses the liver and kidneys, as well as aiding in maintaining a healthy digestive system and regulating appetite. It mainly works by suppressing the appetite and boosting the metabolic rate, which helps weight control.

Cinnamon Tea

Cinnamon tea is not only delicious, but very good for you as it has many health benefits. Cinnamon could regulate blood sugar levels and reduce (LDL) bad cholesterol levels and is excellent for stomach and digestive system health.

Cinnamon tea also has weight loss properties. Be aware that cinnamon tea is not cinnamon and sugar tea! It's the sugar that people put with their cinnamon that negates the weight loss benefits.

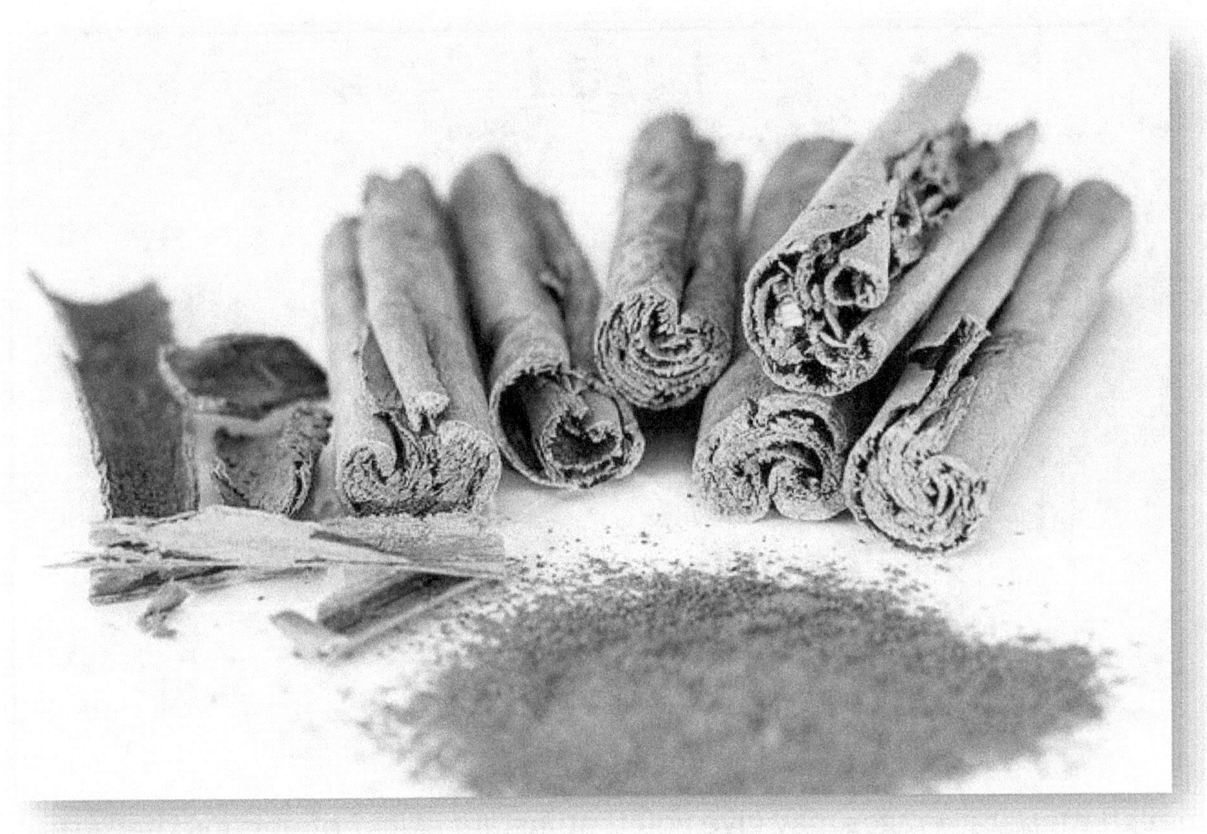

Herbal Teas that Boost Energy

What better way to get a pick-me-up by putting the kettle on! Many, or should we say, most people rely on coffee and other energy drinks whenever they feel like they need a quick boost of energy.

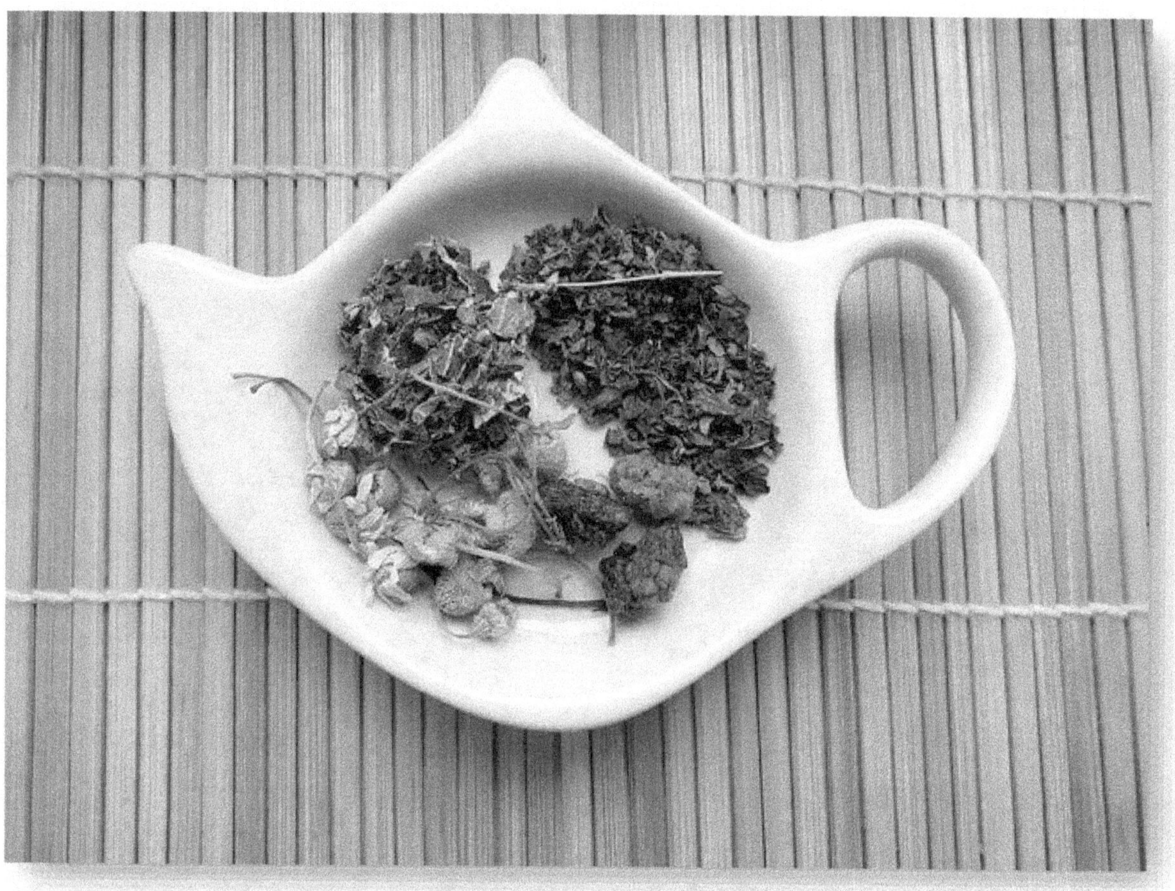

Although these beverages may give you that instant "kick" of energy, they are never without side effects.

The caffeine content of coffee has been found by researchers to put a strain on the adrenal cortex as it is forced to release more energy. However, you can avoid this unhealthy activity by drinking healthier beverages such as herbal teas.

The following are some of the best herbal teas you can have on hand for that instant pick-me-up drink at home, in the workplace or anywhere!

Gingko Biloba Tea

Gingko Biloba is most famous for enhancing memory and is widely given to patients suffering from Alzheimer's disease and dementia. However, it is also beneficial for improving blood circulation and for boosting energy levels. The ability of Gingko Biloba to improve energy, cognition, stamina and motivation can be partly attributed to its high amounts of omega 3 fatty acids.

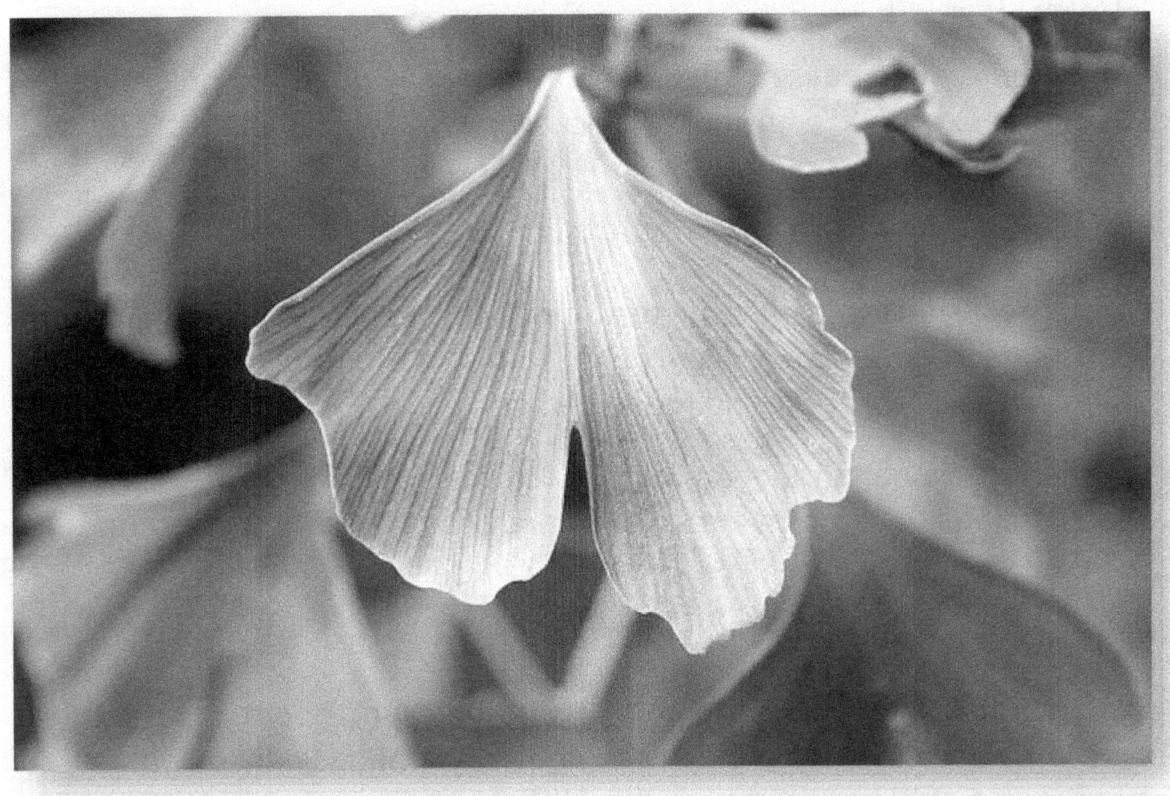

Scientific studies show that Ginkgo Biloba works effectively at increasing blood circulation which provides better oxygen flow through the cells and tissues to the brain. This brings about improved clarity and better focus.

This result is why many people claim that drinking Ginkgo Biloba tea gives them a feeling of alertness. Ginkgo Biloba is also a common ingredient found in many energy drinks today.

By drinking it as a home-made tea, you can reap the benefits without consuming the added sugar and other ingredients which don't contribute to your health.

Korean Ginseng Tea

Korean Ginseng contains adaptogens, which are plant extracts that help the body fight against stress and the damage that stress symptoms can cause to your health. It also provides some of the essential nutrients for the adrenal cortex to function at an optimal level.

Korean Ginseng contains active compounds that provides not only lasting energy, but also stress-resistant energy.

This is something coffee does not provide. Caffeine may provide a quick energy boost, but it doesn't provide any neurological support, so it is not a 'stress-resistant' energy.

Siberian Ginseng Tea

This tea is quite distinct from ginseng tea. Although this herb is called "ginseng" it does not actually belong to the ginseng family. It is another powerful adaptogen herb which helps boost energy and reduce fatigue.

Siberian ginseng also has anti-inflammatory and analgesic effects and has been shown to be helpful in reducing stress levels and strengthening the immune system.

Ashwagandha Tea

This is another adaptogen herb that helps fight fatigue and boost your energy. It also helps reduce anxiety levels, stabilizes blood sugar and lowers blood cholesterol.

Yerba Mate Tea

This herb is known to be an excellent alternative to coffee and energy drinks. Yerba Mate contains properties that are like that of caffeine, however, it doesn't cause sleeping difficulties like coffee does. It gives you a natural energy boost without the side effects.

Yerba Mate has many health benefits. It doesn't just boost energy and fight fatigue, it also helps suppress the appetite, lower bad cholesterol levels (when taken three times a day for a period of 40 days) and a whole lot more!

Health Benefits of Chamomile Tea

This is one of the most popular herbal teas and is one herbal tea that requires more than just a short summary.

Chamomile is the common name of plants that have daisy-like flowers and is derived from a Greek word which means 'earth apple'.

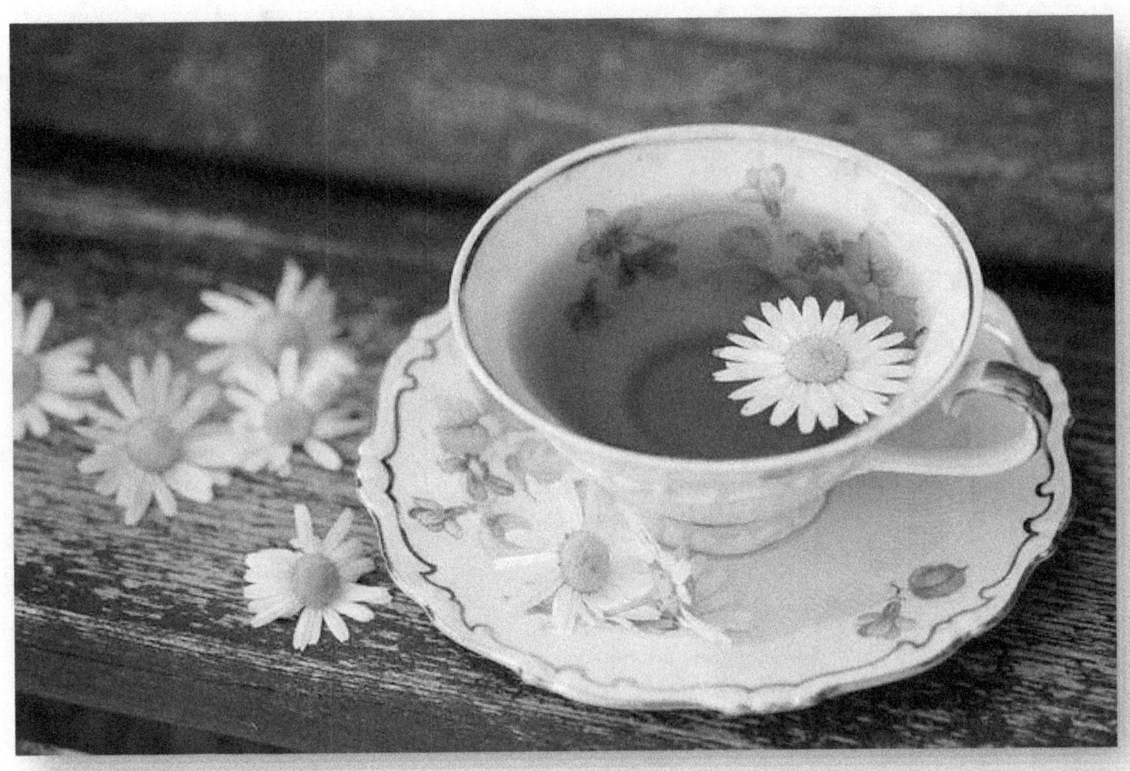

There are many sub-species and it has been widely studied due to its many health benefits. Let's look at a few of the benefits:

Provides a Restful Night's Sleep

Chamomile is well-known for its ability to induce sleep. According to research, chemical compounds have been identified in chamomile which relieves anxiety and relaxes the nervous system, thus making sleep easier.

These chemical compounds function by soothing and refreshing the muscles and the brain, which puts the person in a more relaxed state. To best induce sleep, chamomile tea should be taken 30 to 45 minutes before bed.

Provides Digestive Relief and Support

Chamomile tea aids in soothing indigestion and relieving stomach pains. It helps provide regular bowel movements and alleviates irritable bowel syndrome.

Chamomile tea is also recommended for patients suffering with GERD - gastroesophageal reflux disease - as it helps calm the acid content of the stomach and dispel gas accumulation in the intestines.

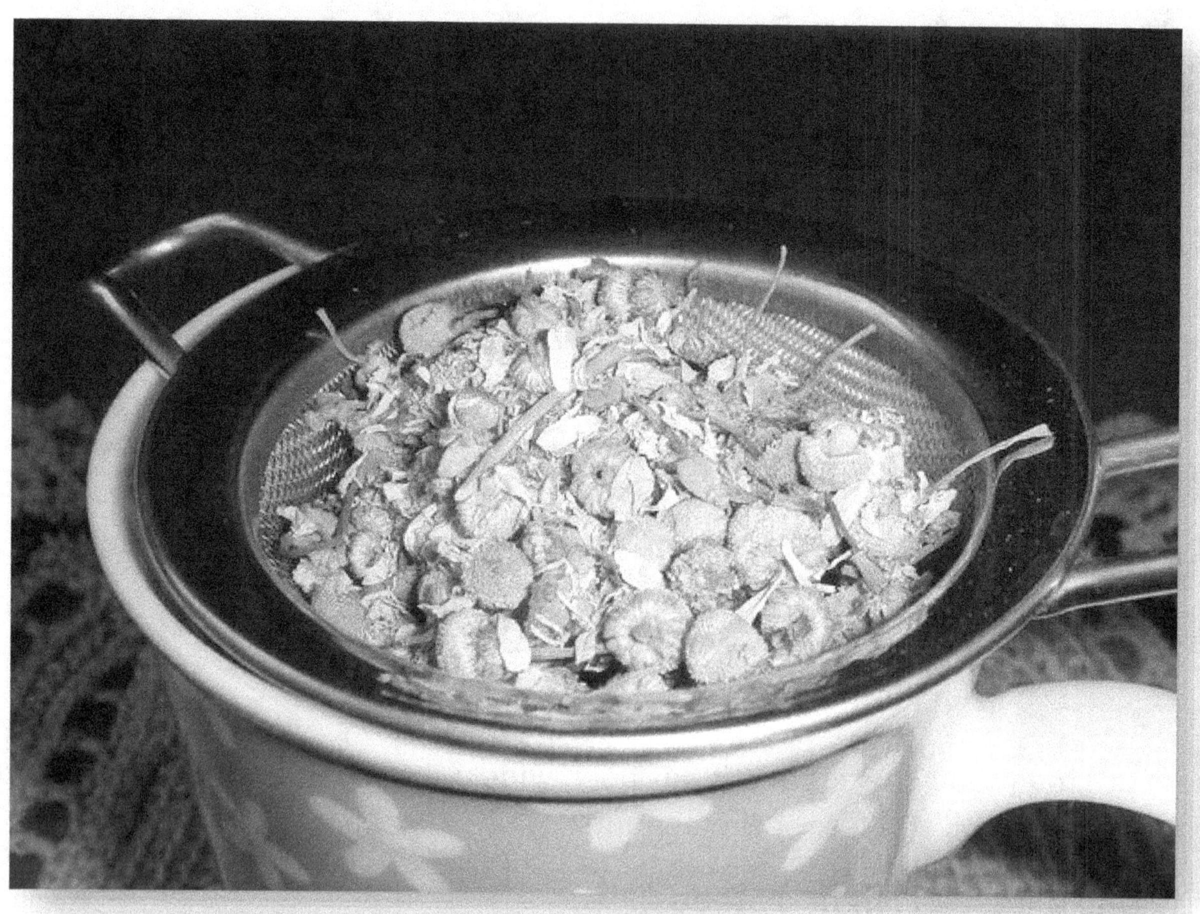

Alleviates Muscle Spasms and Cramps

Ancient Egyptians used chamomile to relieve menstrual cramps, as do women today.

Studies show that chamomile increases the levels of glycine in the body, which greatly alleviates muscle spasms and cramps. In addition, it is also efficient in relieving hemorrhoid discomfort.

Relieves Pain and Fever

Chamomile contains antibacterial and anti-inflammatory properties. This makes it a perfect natural solution for relieving migraines, arthritic pains, colds, flu, fever, and for promoting faster healing of wounds and burns.

Cosmetic 'Skin Lightening' Benefits

Chamomile tea bags can be used for lightening the skin and removing dark circles from around the eyes. To remove dark circles from under the eyes, dip 2 tea bags in warm water for 2 minutes and let the tea bags cool for 5 minutes. Then you can apply them over your eyes.

Relieves Stress and Anxiety

Chamomile tea is used by anxiety sufferers to relieve their anxiousness and promote a sense of calm. Chamomile helps relax the central nervous system and keeps adrenaline hormones from surging, which causes palpitations.

It is also helping relieve stress, fatigue, and irritability. The relaxing and sedative component of chamomile is one of the many reasons that it has been recommended by many holistic practitioners and herbalists all over the world.

Types of Teas and Their Health Benefits

From green tea to hibiscus, from white tea to chamomile, teas are chock full of flavonoids and other healthy goodies.

Regarded for thousands of years in the Far East as a key to good health, happiness, wisdom, sleeping aids, stimulator, tea has caught the attention of researchers in the West, who are discovering the many health benefits of different types of teas. Teas in the orient where used for trade, in place of gold.

Many Ancient and modern studies have found that some teas may help with brain function, heart disease, and diabetes; encourage weight loss; lower cholesterol; and bring about mental alertness. Tea also appears to have antimicrobial qualities. We are only on the verge of finding all the abilities plants must help with so many different mind and organ functions.

"There doesn't seem to be a downside to tea," says the author Cheri DeShaw. I have always drunk tea; coffee was never a choice for me. Saying that: "I think it's a great alternative to coffee drinking. First, most herbal tea has less caffeine. It's been established that the compounds in herbal tea – their flavonoids – are good for the heart and may possibly reduce cancer."

Although a lot of questions remain about how long tea needs to be steeped for the most benefit, and how much you need to drink, nutritionists agree any herbal tea is good tea. I prefer brewed teas over bottled to avoid the extra calories and sweeteners. Myself I use natural sweeteners like honey, date nibs or stevia.

Health Benefits of Tea: Green, Black, and White Tea

Tea is a name given to a lot of brews, but purists consider only green tea, black tea, white tea, oolong tea, and Pu-erh tea the real thing. They are all derived from the *Camellia sinensis* plant, a shrub native to China and India, and contain unique antioxidants called flavonoids. The most potent of these, known as ECGC, may help against free radicals that may contribute to cancer, heart disease, and clogged arteries.

All these teas also have caffeine and theanine, which affect the brain and seem to heighten mental alertness.

The more processed the tea leaves, usually the less polyphenol content. Polyphenols include flavonoids. Oolong and black teas are oxidized or fermented, so they have lower concentrations of polyphenols than green tea; but their antioxidizing power is still high.

Here's what some studies have found about the potential health benefits of tea, these studies can be found in researching on WebMD:

- **Green tea**: Made with steamed tea leaves, it has a high concentration of EGCG and has been widely studied. Green tea's antioxidants may interfere with the growth of bladder, breast, lung, stomach, pancreatic, and colorectal cancers; prevent clogging of the arteries, burn fat, counteract oxidative stress on the brain, reduce risk of neurological disorders like Alzheimer's and Parkinson's diseases, reduce risk of stroke, and improve cholesterol levels.
- **Black tea**: Made with fermented tea leaves, black tea has the highest caffeine content and forms the basis for flavored teas like chai, along with some instant teas. Studies have shown that black tea may protect lungs from damage caused by exposure to cigarette smoke. It also may reduce the risk of stroke.
- **White tea**: Uncured and unfermented. One study showed that white tea has the most potent anticancer properties compared to more processed teas.
- **Oolong tea**: In an animal study, those given antioxidants from oolong tea were found to have lower bad cholesterol levels. One variety of oolong, Wuyi, is heavily marketed as a weight loss supplement, but science hasn't backed the claims.
- **Pu-erh tea**: Made from fermented and aged leaves. Considered a black tea, its leaves are pressed into cakes. One animal study showed that animals given Pu-erh had less weight gain and reduced LDL cholesterol.

It is important to note that you can grow most of these teas in your backyard or greenhouse and pick fresh, dry and use year-round. Peppermint and spearmint are very popular garden teas to grow. Storage of these is an important factor.

Types of Teas and Their Health Benefits

From Green Tea to Hibiscus, from White Tea to Chamomile, all teas are full of flavonoids and wellness properties. Every continent and country has their own collections.

Health Benefits of Tea: Herbal Teas

Made from herbs, fruits, seeds, or roots steeped in hot water, herbal teas have lower concentrations of antioxidants than green, white, black, and oolong teas. Their chemical compositions vary widely depending on the plant used.

Varieties include ginger, ginkgo biloba, ginseng, hibiscus, jasmine, rosehip, mint, rooibos (red tea), chamomile, and echinacea.

Limited research has been done on the health benefits of herbal teas, but claims that they help to shed pounds, stave off colds, and bring on restful sleep are largely unsupported. More and more information is being gathered to record the many ways in which we can use herbs to heal thyself in a natural way.

Here are some findings:

- Chamomile tea: Its antioxidants may help prevent complications from diabetes, like loss of vision and nerve and kidney damage, and stunt the growth of cancer cells.
- Echinacea: Often touted as a way to fight the common cold, the research on echinacea has been inconclusive. Very popular in the alternative market.
- Hibiscus: A small study found that drinking three cups of hibiscus tea daily lowered blood pressure in people with modestly elevated levels.
- Rooibos (red tea): A South African herb that is fermented. Although it has flavonoids with cancer-fighting properties, medical studies have been limited.

Health Benefits of Tea: Instant teas

Instant tea may contain very little amounts of actual tea and plenty of sugars or artificial sweeteners. For health's sake, check out the ingredients on the label.

Not all suppliers or manufacturers of tea are giving you the right information on their labels, they are trying to hype you on the taste, which is important: warning there are 86 different names for sugar: sugar may not be your friend.

All About Herbal Tea

People use herbal teas to relieve many types of health problems. What do these teas look like and what does science say about how well they work? I have gathered the following information from WebMD.

What's the Difference?

True tea -- whether it's black, green, white, or oolong, hot, or iced -- comes from the tea plant, *Camellia sinensis.* But the herbal kind comes from soaking various flowers, leaves, or spices in hot water. Most of these brews don't have caffeine. You can start with premade bags or loose material you steep and then strain out. Herbal teas are also called "tisanes."

Can Tea Be Bad for Your Health?

Most teas are benign, but the FDA has issued warnings about so-called dieter's teas that contain senna, aloe, buckthorn, and other plant-derived laxatives.

The agency also warns consumers to be wary of herb-containing supplements that claim to kill pain and fight cancer. None of the claims is backed by science and some of the herbs have led to bowel problems, liver and kidney damage, and even death.

The FDA cautions against taking supplements that include:

- Comfrey
- Ephedra
- Willow bark
- Germander
- Lobelia
- Chaparral

These cautions aside, nutritionists say to drink up and enjoy the health benefits of tea. Usually when you combine more than one tea types together it may or can lead to issues. Tea is different than supplements you may take yet be aware of your own bodies reactions to anything you take and be sure to check the labels. If you can't pronounce or recognize the ingrediencies, be aware it may be something your body may not need or want. Look it up on the internet.

Rooibos

Native to South Africa, and a drink made from Rooibos is called Red Bush Tea. It's caffeine-free and appears to have many antioxidants and wellness benefits. Connected to boosting the immune system, heart and help fight diabetes, it has a pleasant taste. There is also a green rooibos with similar benefits. When adding a small amount of honey, dates or natural sweetener, it becomes a real delightful evening treat.

Chamomile

For centuries, people have used this flowering plant to ease upset stomach, gas, diarrhea, insomnia, and anxiety. Some research suggests that it may help relieve generalized anxiety disorder, but there's not much evidence to back other claims. You shouldn't drink it if you're allergic to ragweed. It's also known to interact with blood thinners, such as warfarin, as well as some other drugs.

Rose Hip

This drink is made from the seed pods of a wild variety of the flower. The plant is a source of vitamin C and may have anti-inflammatory and antioxidant powers. Some evidence suggests rose hips might ease arthritis pain, but researchers want to study the effects more closely. It's generally safe, though some people have allergic reactions or an upset stomach when they use it.

Peppermint

Upset stomach, headache, irritable bowel syndrome, and breathing problems are some of the reasons people reach for this herb. Drinks made from the leaves have been used medicinally for centuries, but there's little research to back up any health claims. Peppermint oil in pills or that you put on your skin have been studied a bit more, but scientists need to know more about the benefits. But the brew is safe, so there's no harm in giving it a try or just enjoying the cool taste.

Ginger

The drink made from the root of this tropical plant is mainly a treatment for upset stomach and nausea. You might also try it to boost your appetite, to relieve arthritis pain, or to fight a cold. Although some studies show it can fight queasiness, scientists haven't found much proof of other benefits. This herbal tea is safe, but if you're pregnant, you should check with your doctor before you make it a regular part of your diet.

Lemon Balm

Anxious? Trouble sleeping? Folk wisdom says this herb might be just the thing for you, and there's some evidence to back that up. It may also improve memory, although researchers want to learn more. You might find it gives you nausea or belly pain, though, so be careful about getting too much or using it for a long period of time.

Milk Thistle and Dandelion

People use these brews for problems with their liver and gallbladder. Dandelion tea won't harm you -- unless you're allergic to the yellow-flowered weed -- but studies haven't shown that it's helpful, either. The main ingredient in milk thistle is called silymarin, and one study found that it may ease symptoms of hepatitis C. Researchers believe it's safe for most people.

Hibiscus

This flower, which originally came from ancient Egypt, produces a red brew full of antioxidants. Some small studies have found that it can lower blood pressure. Could it also cut cholesterol? It shows promise, but researchers want to investigate it more. As long you as you drink it in moderation, it's considered safe.

Echinacea

Coneflower (its common name) is known as a cold remedy, but science doesn't back that up. It does seem to boost the immune system, and researchers are studying it as a treatment for the flu. If you're pregnant or have allergies or asthma, it's best to steer clear. It can also affect how well certain drugs work.

Sage

People have used this herb for centuries for issues that include stomach problems, sore throats, depression, and memory loss. Will it really help you with any of those? We don't know because there's not much research on it, and the existing studies are flawed. It's safe to use as a spice or seasoning, but some varieties have an ingredient, thujone, that can affect your nervous system.

Passionflower

Some say this wildflower eases anxiety and helps you sleep, and some research supports those claims. You shouldn't drink the tea if you're pregnant. It can affect the way some medicines work, including pentobarbital and benzodiazepines. It might also cause drowsiness, dizziness, and confusion.

Turmeric

It comes from a root that's related to ginger. People use it to prevent gas and to treat kidney stones, though there's no scientific basis for any of that. Studies in animals show that it may help prevent cancer and reduce inflammation, but researchers need to investigate those effects in humans. If you're getting chemotherapy, you should know this herb may interfere with your treatment.

Valerian

Women use this plant to relieve symptoms of menopause, and you might also take it for insomnia, anxiety, or depression. It hasn't been studied much, so scientists can't really say whether it helps these conditions. Some research suggests it might help you sleep. It's generally safe to use it for a short period of time, but because it might make you sleepy, don't mix it with alcohol or sedatives.

Kava

This member of the pepper family, native to the South Pacific, is often promoted as a tonic for anxiety. Researchers have found that it may give a little relief for that condition, but they've also uncovered links to severe liver problems. People who drink a lot of it for a long time may have yellow or dry, scaly skin. The FDA has issued warnings about the risks of this plant, and some countries have tried to remove it from the market.

What Is Matcha? Green Tea

It's a form of green tea that's been enjoyed in China and Japan for hundreds of years. The leaves are made into a powder that's far stronger than regular tea, so a little can go a long way. Antioxidants are substances in foods that can help protect your cells from damage. Some studies show that because of the way it's made, matcha may have more of those than loose-leaf green tea. Lower Blood Pressure Catechins, an antioxidant in matcha, may help with this. They seem to be especially helpful if your upper number is 130 or higher, which can raise your chances of heart disease, heart attack, and stroke, among other issues.

Alchemy and Tea

I have been a tea drinker for over 50 years, traveled the world and tried various teas from every continent. Over the last 30 years I have indulged more in the **Chemistry of Tea** and the **healing properties**. On the following pages you will find the most beneficial teas for various ailments, including many herbs and other ingrediencies that enhance the flavor and taste. There is a chemistry to tea, and it has been used in every religion from around the world. Rituals are very common in various parts of the world for celebration and the healing properties along with proper combinations to reach a desired quality of product. Many different groups of people, mainly the herbalists, shamans, chemists, native americans, asians, church groups consider some of their combination of all natures herbs to be able to cure the disease's that are recognized in modern times.

I was raised in the NW with an Alchemist as a father and a great grandmother that was familiar with many different herb combinations for most every ailment. Discover on the following pages what might meet your needs.

More Healthy Teas

In addition to the herbal teas already discussed, there are plenty of others. Here are a many more of the ancient and better-known herbal teas, a brief summary of their health benefits and how they can be used to treat certain conditions or ailments.

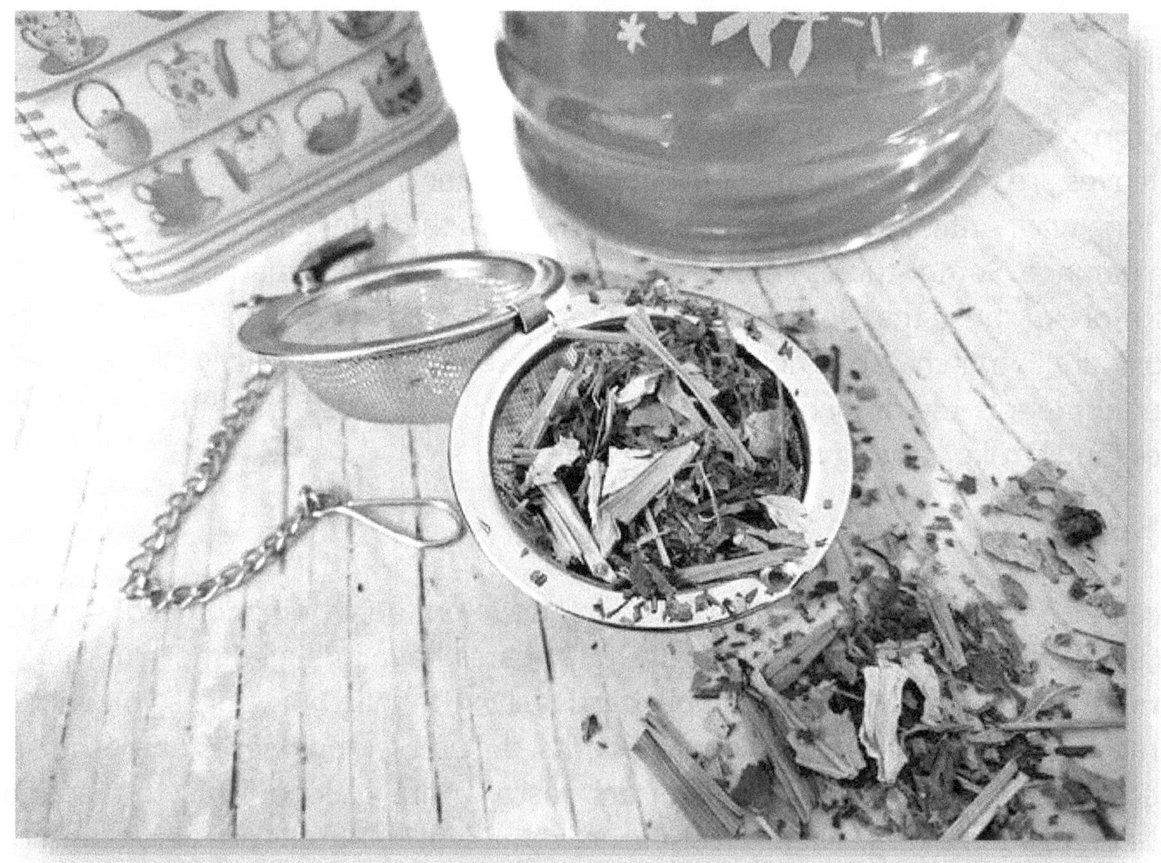

Sage Tea

Sage tea is useful for treating colds, flu, sore throat, menstrual cramps, pain, inflammation and easing menopausal symptoms. It can also aid in digestion and promotes weight loss and hair growth.

Peppermint Tea

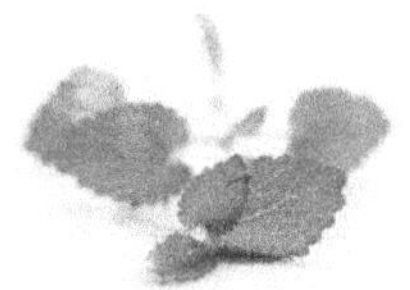

This tea contains no caffeine, yet it improves concentration and focus, to help get through the day's tasks more efficiently. It does not cause mental agitation, which caffeine can, but helps to reduce stress and encourage clear, calm thought.

It is effective in relieving digestive problems, menstrual cramps, sinus problems and headaches. Peppermint tea can help weight loss goals by suppressing appetite and increasing metabolism.

Ginger Tea

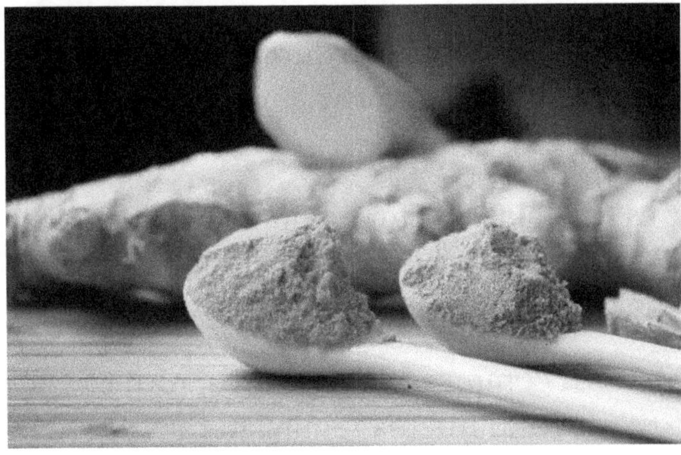

Ginger tea makes use of the ginger root or rhizome and is very famous in Asia for its calming and soothing effects. Ginger tea improves the immune system, enhances blood flow and helps maintain normal circulation, reduces pain and inflammation, relieves morning sickness and nausea, and relieves abdominal discomfort.

Rosemary Tea

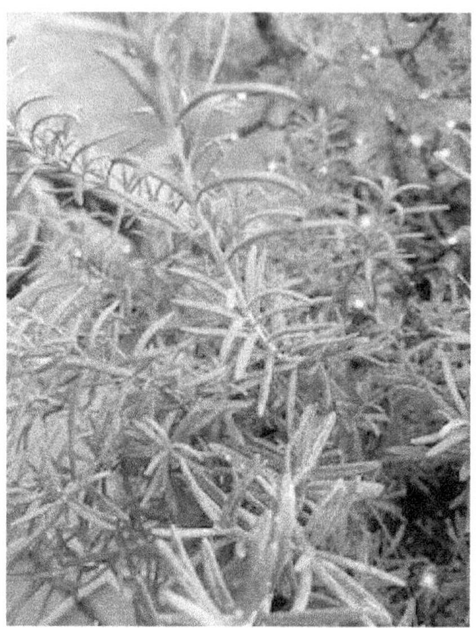

This is a picture of one of my Rosemary plants. I decorate up during the holidays and have it in Palm Springs on my deck. I grow this plant most anywhere I've lived over the last 70 years. Great fragrance to add to the season.

This herb has natural antibiotic properties that aids in fighting off colds, flu and headaches. It contains antioxidants and vitamins that boosts the immune system and helps fight off invading organisms that can cause sickness.

Now that we have looked at some of the most common plants, herbs, roots, berries, spices, sweeteners that go into to teas and the tea family, here is a further reference to help understand. Enjoy your search.

Pages 27 thru 56 provide you with an alphabetic list of useful herbs for tea and their benefits, as collected from various sources and internet such as WebMD, Google Search and Amazon. It is a collection of information I've gathered over a total of 50 years. If you have more information that you feel would be helpful for others please email me at TheSpiritedAlchemy@gmail.com for a revision to be updated in years to come.

Aloe Vera

- Contains healthful plant compounds. Share on Pinterest. ...
- Antioxidant and antibacterial properties. ...
- Accelerates the healing of burns. ...
- Reduces dental plaque. ...
- Helps treat canker sores. ...
- Reduces constipation. ...
- May improve skin and prevent wrinkles. ...
- Lowers blood sugar levels.

Constipation and digestive distress, moisturizer, parasite purge, radiation burns, skin surgery, sunburn. Gel is used from the leaves.

Acai Berries

Acai berries have an incredibly high number of antioxidants, edging out other antioxidant-rich fruits like blueberries and cranberries. In the case of acai, 100 grams of frozen pulp has an ORAC of 15,405, whereas the same number of blueberries has a score of 4,669. Improve cholesterol levels. Brain function, possible anti-cancer.

African Pygeum

- What is pygeum? ...
- It may help treat benign prostatic hyperplasia (BPH) ...
- It may help treat prostate cancer. ...
- It may help treat prostatitis symptoms. ...
- It may help reduce general inflammation. ...
- It may help treat symptoms of kidney disease. ...
- It may help treat urinary conditions. ...
- It may help treat symptoms of malaria

Shown to improve prostate function. Male health.

Angelica Root

Angelica is used for heartburn (dyspepsia), intestinal gas (flatulence), loss of appetite (anorexia), overnight urination (nocturia), arthritis, stroke, dementia, circulation problems, "runny nose" (respiratory catarrh), nervousness and anxiety, fever, plague, and trouble sleeping (insomnia) Chi energy, digestive regulator, antiviral, antifungal and fights bacteria, heart and blood tonic, liver, muscles, nerves, women's menopause. Avoid if diabetic.

Apples

Apples add flavor to your teas and can help with your digestion track. Apples promote heart health in several ways. They're high in soluble fiber, which helps lower cholesterol. They also have polyphenols, which are linked to lower blood pressure and stroke risk. Nutritious, weight loss, asthma, bone health, diabetics.

Apple Cider

Apple cider tea is known to have overall health benefits for common ailments, detoxification, digestive issues, sore throat, weight loss and bad breath, along with having a soothing taste.

Artichoke Leaf

Here are the top 8 health benefits of artichokes and artichoke extract.

- Loaded with Nutrients. ...
- May Lower 'Bad' LDL Cholesterol and Increase 'Good' HDL Cholesterol. ...
- May Help Regulate Blood Pressure. ...
- May Improve Liver Health. ...
- May Improve Digestive Health. ...
- May Ease Symptoms of Irritable Bowel Syndrome. ...
- May Help Lower Blood Sugar.

Aronia Berry

Researchers believe that aronia berries may have protective effects on the liver, as well as helping to reduce symptoms and damage associated with stomach disorders. Finally, aronia seems to be effective in reducing blood pressure and aiding blood vessel relaxation. Heart Health, Longevity, Antioxidants.

Ashwagandha

Natural Menopause Relief - Whatever Stage You're In - Improve Mood, Sleep & Energy

- Is an ancient medicinal herb. ...
- Can reduce blood sugar levels. ...
- Might have anticancer properties. ...
- Can reduce cortisol levels. ...
- May help reduce stress and anxiety. ...
- May reduce symptoms of depression. ...
- Can boost testosterone and increase fertility in men. ...
- May increase muscle mass and strength.

Astragalus Root

A root tea with amino acids to restore your immunity and maintain strong defenses. It also can be used to enhance other teas

Avocado Leaves

Helps lower blood pressure, reduces anxiety, promotes gut health.

Basil

Holy **basil** along with Basil has been shown to reduce stress, treat ulcers, relieve joint pain, and more. Basil has many different health benefits.

Bee Pollen

Bee pollen—your best friend. A powerful and easily assimilated source of B vitamins, minerals, free forming amino acids, and protein, raw bee pollen provides powerful energy support. This superfood is fantastic for anyone leading an on-the-go lifestyle and looking for a tasty infusion of energizing nutrients.

Bilberries

Has been known to fight inflammation, improve vision, lower blood sugar levels, improve brain function, kill bacteria, improve symptoms of ulcerative colitis (UC)

Bitter Melon

Blood sugar control, Test-tube studies show that bitter melon may have cancer-fighting properties and could be effective against stomach, colon, lung, nasopharynx, and breast cancer cells. Decrease cholesterol levels, aid in weight loss. Also known as Bitter Gourd.

Black Cohosh

Natural hormone balance, menopause, has been found to reduce vaginal dryness and hot flashes in menopausal women.

Black Currants

- blood flow
- immune system
- eye health
- gut health
- kidney health

Black Pepper

High in antioxidants, has anti-inflammatory properties. May benefit your brain, improve blood sugar control, lower cholesterol levels, have cancer-fighting properties, boosts absorption of nutrients, promote gut health, offer pain relief, reduce appetite.

Blue Berries (Flavor)

Picked, dried in the sun and infused with boiling water, blackberry leaves are the essence of most berry-flavored teas. Studies suggest that the leaves contain a healthy dose of flavonoids, which are known for their antioxidant activity. Enhance other tea ingrediencies.

Blue Corn Flower

Cornflower blossoms contain anthocyanins (main component: succinyl cyanine), flavonoids and bitter substances. Cornflower blossoms are used in natural healing as herbal tea or in ointments.

Bur Marigold Oil or Leaves

This oil extract is actively used in cosmetology to cease itching and inflammation of the skin. It improves skin condition with diathesis, neurodermatitis and skin rashes. It is an excellent tool for strengthening dry and brittle hair - for this effect it is necessary to put oil on the scalp, rub lightly, leaving for 30 minutes, then rinsing. Also used for preparation of medicinal baths. It is widely used in pediatric practice.

Cacao husks Blend

Full of antioxidants - Cacao contains theobromine, a molecule responsible for our well-being, but also that facilitates blood circulation and reduces stress.

Carrot Juice (Pure)

Increased metabolism, stronger vision, improve skin disorders, boosted immune system, reduced cancer risk, lowered cholesterol, healthier pregnancy, strengthened brain function.

Catnip

Catnip tea's biggest health benefit is the calming effect that it can have on the body. Catnip contains nepetalactone, which is like the valepotriates found in a commonly used herbal sedative, valerian. This can improve relaxation, which may boost mood and reduce anxiety, restlessness, and nervousness. Cat's love it and want to be close to it.

Catnip tea can stimulate uterine contractions, which can help women or girls with delayed menstruation get their periods. It may also help promote evacuations of the placenta following childbirth.

Calendula

Calendula is also known as pot marigold. It's a centuries-old antifungal, antiseptic, wound-healing ally.

Cardamom

High blood pressure, May Contain Cancer-Fighting Compounds, protect from chronic diseases thanks to anti-Inflammatory effects, help with digestive problems, including ulcers, treat bad breath and prevent cavities, have antibacterial effects and treat infections, improve breathing and oxygen use, lower blood sugar levels, liver protection, anxiety, weight loss.

Cayenne Pepper

Promotes Cardiovascular Health, detox, Joints, preserve food from bacteria anti-redness properties, helps produce saliva, heart health, longevity, anti-irritant properties, clears congestion, headache remedy, digestive aid, topical remedy, toothache, also known to help rid yourself of some types of parasites.

Celery Root

Celeriac is packed with antioxidants, which are anti-inflammatory , they may work by fighting against harmful free radicals, thus protecting healthy cells from damage. In doing so, they may protect against many conditions, such as heart disease, cancer and Alzheimer's. They may even offer anti-aging effects.

Chamomile

A floral tea to help unwind at night. It eases stomachaches, soothes your nerves and lulls you into sleep. It also fights E. coli.

Chamomile is a flower long loved for its soothing, calming and sleep-inducing qualities. The petals of the plant are the active ingredient—and are most often combined with other soothing herbs like valerian and hops to create the blends meant to lull you into relaxation, sleep or naps.

Chaste Berry

Chasteberry Fruit, also known as Vitex agnus- castus, has a long history of use by women during their periods. Studies suggest that it has a progesterone-like effect, which may account for its use in the support of women's health. Because of this activity, chasteberry has been recommended for a variety of issues common to PMS including mood, body tenderness and water balance.

Cherries

Cherries are a great source of bioactive compounds known as anthocyanins, which may have anti-inflammatory, anti-cancer, and cardiovascular benefits. Sleep benefits, ease achy joints.

Chicory Root

Digestive, heart, oral, sodium reduction, low sugar, increase protein.

Cocoa Husks

Cacao shells have been found to make a superb cup of tea, thanks to its delicious flavor and phenomenal health benefits. Cacao shells are packed with antioxidants, amino acids, magnesium, iron, and zinc. Enjoy this healthy herbal tea for the perfect dessert alternative.

Cinnamon Bark

Cinnamon bark powder is extracted from the cinnamon tree, specifically from the Cinnamomic wilsonii tree. Rich in antioxidant and anti-inflammatory compounds, it may benefit heart and cognitive health.

Ceylon (Green)

Ceylon Teas Benefits

- Weight Loss. Ceylon teas can help you lose weight. ...
- Heart Health. Ceylon teas contain potassium. ...
- Chronic Diseases. The antioxidants in Ceylon teas can help prevent many chronic diseases. ...
- Diabetes. ...
- Skin Care. ...
- Energy Boost. ...
- Kidney Health. ...
- Bone Health.

Green Tea has too long of a list for health benefits. I drink it every day. This tea has been recognized in the USA as a healthy substitute for replacing coffee. It is combined with many different herbal ingredients and is available in most every Starbucks or Coffee shops in the USA.

Cloves

8 Health Benefits of Cloves

1. Contain Important Nutrients.
2. High in Antioxidants. ...
3. May Protect Against Cancer. ...
4. Can Kill Off Bacteria. ...
5. May Improve **Liver** Health. ...
6. May Help Regulate Blood Sugar. ...
7. May Promote Bone Health. ...
8. May Reduce Stomach Ulcers.

A spice or herb for year-round. A great delight to any tea for great flavor and taste. Smells great during the holidays, I use it with orange peel.

Cranberries

Many people consider cranberries to be a superfood due to their high nutrient and antioxidant content. In fact, some research has linked the nutrients in cranberries to a possible lower risk of urinary tract infection (UTI), the prevention of certain types of cancer, improved immune function, and decreased blood pressure. A berry tea for vitamin C, B-complex, iron, and calcium—the antistressor nutrients. Also cleanses the urinary tract, bladder, and kidney.

Dandelion Leaf or Dandelion Root

Dandelion root tea can have many positive effects on your digestive system, although much of the evidence is anecdotal. It has historically been used to improve appetite, soothe minor digestive ailments, and possibly relieve constipation. A root or leaf for toning your liver and removing toxins. It's natural diuretic with potassium to maintain electrolyte balance. Grows freely in the USA.

Dried Dates

According to TCM, red dates help replenish and nourish your blood, thus improving blood circulation. This can lead to better liver and digestive function, balance of inner body energy and improved immunity. Pitted dates are Mother Earth's all-natural sweetener. Edible energy, replenish potassium, fabulous for fiber.

Dark Chocolate nips or Dark Chocolate Chips

Relieve stress, lower blood pressure, lower cholesterol, brain function, aids weight loss, number of antioxidants, chocolate will almost entirely neutralize the effects of free radicals. Flavonoids in the chocolate can help your skin get protection from ultraviolet sun rays.

Echinacea

A root tea for colds, flues, infections, gland swelling and inflammation. It can also be used as a topical wash for skin infections. Used as a tincture.

There is much debate over whether echinacea really prevents or cures the common cold. But it's widely acknowledged as a powerful herb that contains active substances that may enhance the activity of the immune system, relieve pain, reduce inflammation and have antioxidant effects. The tea is prepared by infusing with hot water the leaves and flowers of the uppermost part of the plant—the section believed to contain polysaccharides (a substance known to trigger the activity of the immune system).

Elderberry

Elderberries are rich in antioxidants and minerals. Their rich antioxidants make them perfect in battling the common cold. Great to enhance the immune system. Like elderflower properties.

Elderflower

Elderflower is the flower of a tree. An extract of the flower is used to make wellness products and medicine. Can be used for swollen sinuses (sinusitis), colds, influenza (flu), swine flu, bronchitis, diabetes, and constipation. It is also used to increase urine production (as a diuretic), to increase sweating (as a diaphoretic), and to stop bleeding.
Elderflower is also used as a gargle and mouthwash for coughs, colds, hoarseness (laryngitis), flu, and shortness of breath. It is used on the skin for joint pain (rheumatism), and pain and swelling (inflammation).
Some people put elderflower in the eyes for red eyes. Great for teas.

Eyebright

A tea for the computer age, the whole plant eases eyestrain, lifts your spirits, clears your head, and gives you a very clear focus. Great after working a long day and wanting a refreshing look for head and vison clarity.

Eucalyptus leave

They may help decrease pain, promote relaxation, and relieve cold symptoms. Many over-the-counter products also use eucalyptus extract to freshen your breath, soothe irritated skin, and repel insects. Eucalyptus tea is considered safe to drink, but ingesting eucalyptus oil can be toxic in relatively low doses. Mainly known for lung and respiratory issues. Be cautious, I have a reaction to eucalyptus leaves and I'm not able to drink tea or have leaves or trees around me.

Fennel Seed

- SUPPORTS HEALTHY DIGESTION – May help the smooth muscles of the gastrointestinal system, relaxing them while reducing discomfort.
- FENNEL TEA - COOLING SPICE – Mostly used to treat common stomach discomfort, bloating, gas, cramps, and is effective for treating indigestion.
- LOW CALORIES & HIGHLY NUTRITIOUS – Clean sourced funnel seeds are diet friendly and contain wholesome minerals and vitamins essential to your overall health and wellness.

Fenugreek

* Keep the bowels regular and the digestive system functioning properly
* To neutralize the effect of free radical damage
* Cardiovascular health support
* Support healthy skin, brain health and nervous system
* Lactation Support
* Women's Health
* Anti-Inflammatory and Antioxidant Nutritional Support

Gingko Leaf

- BRAIN HEALTH SUPPORT: Known as the 'brain herb', it is frequently added to nutrition bars, soft drinks, teas and fruit smoothies to support cognitive performance. Studies have shown that ginkgo improves blood circulation by opening blood vessels and making blood less sticky.
- SUPPORTS BLOOD CIRCULATION: Ginkgo Biloba reduces the risk of blood clots by increasing the blood flow to the brain. The blood flow also reduces the chances of free- radical damage of brain cells.
- PROMOTES A HEALTHY VISION: Ginkgo Biloba has been linked to supporting healthy vision in a few research studies.
- ASSISTS WITH GENERAL MOBILITY: Published studies reveal that for certain elderly patients with limited mobility, taking ginkgo biloba helped them walk roughly 37 yards more than simply taking a placebo.

Ginger

- Increase metabolism and support weight loss
- Boost the immune system and fight off disease
- Treat unsightly blemishes, scars, and sunburns
- Promote healthy skin, hair, and nail.

Ginseng

- Boosts energy levels, fights fatigue.
- Defeats stress.
- Encourages mental sharpness.
- Promotes overall body function and balance.
- Supports sexual vitality.
- Excellent for an active lifestyle.

Grape Leaves

Oregon grape is also useful to treat colds, flu, and numerous infections.

Vitamins A, and C, riboflavin, niacin, folate, pantothenic acid, and thiamine.

Oregon Grape Root

The golden yellow root of Oregon grape is commonly harvested as a medicine, and is sometimes substituted for goldenseal, as the two herbs have similar constituent properties. Oregon grape has been clinically shown to support certain skin irritation when used externally. It is also traditionally used as a bitter tonic to stimulate digestion and externally for its antimicrobial properties. The active constituents in Oregon grape root have shown substantial antimicrobial and antifungal activity in vitro, though these activities are unproven in human trials.

Green Rooibos

The attribute that makes this tea an unusual variety when compared to Red Rooibos tea, is that it is completely unfermented, it contains a slightly herbal aftertaste, and brews light in color which makes it a perfect companion to those that feel regular Rooibos is too sweet. Green Rooibos is a hearty tea and once brewed it produces a soft golden color with an amber hue, and warm scent. This tea is considerably higher in antioxidants, trace minerals, and nutrients, when compared to traditional Rooibos, which helps to explain its explosive popularity with those of us who are health conscious.

Guava Leaves

GUAVA LEAF TEA - BLOCKS CARBS BURNS FAT - BLOOD SUGAR SUPPORT - HAIR GROWTH, SKIN SUPPORT - ANTI-AGING ANTIOXIDANTS - ORGANIC, NON-GMO.

Gunpowder Green Tea

- Uplifting, Increases Mental Awareness and Focus
- Powerful Antioxidant, Anti-Aging
- Increases Endurance
- Increases Metabolism and Helps with Weight Loss
- Reduces Cholesterol
- Calorie-free, Fat-free, Gluten-free

Gui Pi Won

Gui Pi Wan (Gui Pi Pian, Gui Pi Tang) is a regarded Chinese herbal formula that strengthens the Spleen and the Heart. It is used to nourish the Blood, replenish Qi, and calm the mind in cases of overwork or stress.

Hawthorn Berries

The leaves, flowers and berries of the hawthorn plant are used in a variety of peach- and berry-flavored teas. The plant is believed to contain flavonoid-like complexes that help improve cardiovascular health by helping to relax and dilate blood vessels, which increases blood circulation and lessens stress on the heart. Hawthorn berries are also believed to relieve water retention by draining the body of excess salt.

Hibiscus

Hibiscus—better known to us as the "zinger" in teas, is an herb favored for its tangy flavor and known health value as a natural diuretic. Great taste.

Honey

Has so many benefits, other than for diabetes, since it can work against your sugar intake system. It has an excellent taste for sweetening your teas. Honey enhanced with Shungite has proven many elevated health benefits. Benefits have been acknowledged from Shungite being used for generating a highly effective honey when place at the entrance of Beehives. I use Shungite honey daily and for any cuts, scratches as a fast wound healing ointment.

Honeybush (Green)

Honeybush is gaining popularity as a caffeine-free alternative to decaffeinated teas. This unoxidized version, which is higher in antioxidants than traditional Honeybush, has an invigorating aroma and flavor notes of citrus and sweet apricot.

Honey Suckle

Honeysuckle is used for digestive disorders including pain and swelling (inflammation) of the small intestine (enteritis) and dysentery; upper respiratory tract infections including colds, influenza, swine flu, and pneumonia; other viral and bacterial infections; swelling of the brain (encephalitis); fever; boils; and sores. Honeysuckle is also used for urinary disorders, headache, diabetes, rheumatoid arthritis, and cancer. Some people use it to promote sweating, as a laxative, to counteract poisoning, and for birth control.
Honeysuckle is sometimes applied to the skin for inflammation and itching, and to kill germs.

Holy Basil

Holy basil, commonly referred to as tulsi, is classified as a perennial plant originally grown in India. Although it is native to India, holy basil is known to grow in other countries around the world today, including Australia, some countries located in the Middle East, and even West Africa. In addition to this, holy basil is known for its aromatic properties. These properties give holy basil multiple uses when it comes to health, both when it is ingested (such as in tea) or when it is applied topically.

Hops

Other benefits of hop **tea** as medicine include the fact that they are high in antioxidants, they are phytoestrogen, antiviral and antimicrobial, anti-carcinogenic, and may help in the treatment of diabetes symptoms. Can relieve sleep and stress issues

Hyssop Herb

It is an expectorant, sedative and anti-spasmodic so it can calm the chest and aid breathing when congested. It combines well with white horehound in the treatment of coughs and chest problems, and with peppermint for the common cold. Digestive system support. Works to revitalize the body, promoting overall wellness

Jasmine

Jasminum sambac—a species of the genus Jasmine (a shrub or vine in the olive family)—is the flower featured in tea blends. Unlike other herbs, jasmine is most loved for its robust fragrance rather than its health value. Typically, the oils from the petals of the flower are combined with a green tea or roobios tea to create the steaming concoction we enjoy.

Kava Kava

Some people take kava by mouth to calm anxiety, stress, and restlessness, and to treat sleeping problems (insomnia). It is also used for attention deficit-hyperactivity disorder (ADHD), withdrawal from benzodiazepine drugs, epilepsy, psychosis, depression, migraines and other headaches, chronic fatigue syndrome (CFS), common cold and other respiratory tract infections, tuberculosis, muscle pain, and cancer prevention.
Some people also take kava by mouth for urinary tract infections (UTIs), pain and swelling of the uterus, venereal disease, menstrual discomfort, and to increase sexual desire.
Kava is applied to the skin for skin diseases including leprosy, to promote wound healing, and as a painkiller. It is also used as a mouthwash for canker sores and toothaches.
Kava is also consumed as a beverage in ceremonies to promote relaxation.

Licorice Root

Gastrointestinal health, menopause, instead of hormone replacement therapy, immune system supporting properties, benefits against harmful organisms.

Lemon

It's all that vitamin C, which is also known as ascorbic acid, Thiamin and riboflavin, part of a group of vitamins called B complex, turn your food into the energy you need, Vitamin C, flavonoids, phenolic acids, essential oils, and coumarins are all plentiful in lemons. Disinfectant, antibiotic, colds, flu to name a few.

Lemon Balm

Anxious? Trouble sleeping? Folk wisdom says this herb might be just the thing for you, and there's some evidence to back that up. It may also improve memory, although researchers want to learn more. You might find it gives you nausea or belly pain, though, so be careful about getting too much or using it for a long period of time.

Lemon Grass

The citrusy tang that comes from the lemongrass plant is favored in cooking as well as tea. Lemongrass teas are often served as an after-dinner drink to aid digestion—primarily due to a substance called citral, also the active ingredient in lemon peels. Though typically enjoyed unaccompanied by other herbs, it can also be blended to create lemon-flavored teas.

Lemon Oil

It's all that vitamin C, which is also known as ascorbic acid, Thiamin and riboflavin, part of a group of vitamins called B complex, turn your food into the energy you need, Vitamin C, flavonoids, phenolic acids, essential oils, and coumarins are all plentiful in lemons. Disinfectant, antibiotic, colds, flu to name a few.

Lemon Peel

It's all that vitamin C, which is also known as ascorbic acid, Thiamin and riboflavin, part of a group of vitamins called B complex, turn your food into the energy you need, Vitamin C, flavonoids, phenolic acids, essential oils, and coumarins are all plentiful in lemons. Disinfectant, antibiotic, colds, flu to name a few.

Lemon Verbena

Lemon Verbena is a stomachic and therefore good for relieving indigestion, heartburn, and for tonifying the digestive tract. It is also great for soothing anxiety and as a sedative it is helpful in insomnia.

Licorice Root

Licorice root is used to soothe gastrointestinal problems. In cases of food poisoning, stomach ulcers, and heartburn, licorice root extract can speed the repair of stomach lining and restore balance. This is due to the anti-inflammatory and immune-boosting properties of glycyrrhizic acid.

Mango

Here are 8 benefits of mango leaves that you may know.

- Regulates Diabetes. Mango leaves are very useful for managing diabetes.
- Lowers blood pressure.
- Fights restlessness.
- Treats gall and kidney stones.
- Treat respiratory problems.
- Treats dysentery.
- Home Remedy for earaches.
- Heals skin burns.

Maple

Maple. Like tea, certain components of the maple tree contain flavonoids. There are high quantities of these molecules in plants, vegetables, and fruits. They protect against heart disease and have antioxidant properties.

Maca Root

There is a range of potential benefits of maca root:

- Increasing libido.
- Reducing erectile dysfunction.
- Boosting energy and endurance.
- Increasing fertility.
- Improving mood.
- Lowering blood pressure.
- Reducing sun damage.
- Fighting free radicals.

Milk Thistle

Seven potential health benefits of milk thistle:

- Supports liver health. One of the most common uses of milk thistle is to treat liver problems.
- Promotes skin health.
- Reduces cholesterol.
- Supports weight loss.
- Reduces insulin resistance.
- Improves allergic asthma symptoms.
- Supports bone health.

Mamaki

Mamaki Properties with Possible Health Benefits

- Catechins – helps to fight diseases and cell damage.
- Chlorogenic acid – help with blood pressure.
- Rutin – helps control bodyweight.

Moringa Leaf

 Studies show that Moringa oleifera may lead to modest reductions in blood sugar and cholesterol. It may also have antioxidant and anti-inflammatory effects and protect against arsenic toxicity. Moringa leaves are also highly nutritious and should be beneficial for people who are lacking in essential nutrients.

Nettle Leaf

Stinging nettle leaf is a gentle diuretic, helping the body to process and flush away toxins. It flushes the kidneys and bladder to prevent and soothe urinary tract infections. Nettle tea is ideal for sodium induced water retention and high blood pressure.

This herbal tea is also rich in Vitamin C and antioxidants. Nettle tea induces weight loss by detoxifying the body and suppressing cravings and appetite.

Oranges and Orange Peel, Orange Pulp

The zest of an orange peel is often the basis of orange, clementine, honey and tangerine teas. It may be unpleasant to eat in its natural state, but when dried and infused with boiling water, the peel produces a strong, aromatic flavor and is known for its immune system–boosting properties.

Olive Leaves

Olive leaf extract

- reduces cardiovascular risk, like atherosclerosis.
- lowers blood pressure.
- helps treats type 2 diabetes.
- supports weight loss.
- eliminates free radicals.
- boosts immunity.
- fights herpes.
- reduces inflammation.

Oregon Basil

Imagine being able to tackle stress, anxiety, and inflammation with a relaxing cup of tea made with the leaves of holy basil. As an adaptogen with anti-inflammatory and antioxidant properties, holy basil provides all these benefits. It can even help people with arthritis or fibromyalgia.

Oregano

6 Science-Based Health Benefits of Oregano

- Rich in Antioxidants.
- May Help Fight Bacteria. Oregano contains certain compounds that have potent antibacterial properties.
- Could Have Anti-Cancer Properties. Oregano is high in antioxidants.
- May Help Reduce Viral Infection.
- Could Decrease Inflammation.
- Easy to Add to Your Diet. Great spice adds flavor.

Passionflower

Incarnate has many common names, including purple passionflower and maypop. Early studies suggest it might help relieve insomnia and anxiety. It appears to boost the level of gamma-aminobutyric acid (GABA) in your brain. This compound lowers brain activity, which may <u>help you relax and sleep better.</u>

Peaches

Here are seven surprising health benefits and uses of peaches.

- Packed with Nutrients and Antioxidants.
- May Aid Digestion.
- May Improve Heart Health.
- May Protect Your Skin.
- May Prevent Certain Types of Cancer.
- May Reduce Allergy Symptoms.
- Widely Available and Easy to Add to Your Tea. Great flavor.

Peppermint and Peppermint Oil

Known as a cure-all, it's a tea for instant energy. The whole plant eases pain, headaches, and tension. A great tea to take on a journey in a thermos, reduces stress without putting you to sleep.

Often peppermint tea is either a mixture of black or green tea with peppermint leaves, or a simple peppermint tisane (sometimes referred to as mint tea). It's believed that the menthol-containing leaves help soothe irritable bowel syndrome, nausea and other stomach-related ailments by calming the abdominal muscles and improving the flow of bile, which aids in digestion. Peppermint is also said to cure minor cases of bad breath and gums.

Plantain-Tea

A leaf tea that detoxifies your blood and is a decongestant for mucus membranes.
It's an excellent tea to keep on hand for emergencies--- in case of poisoning or
toxic conditions. To clean wounds, can be used to wash or compress.

Pumpkin Seed

Here are the top 8 health benefits of pumpkin seeds that are recognized:

- Full of Valuable Nutrients.
- High in Antioxidants.
- Linked to a Reduced Risk of Certain Cancers.
- Improve Prostate and Bladder Health.
- Very High in Magnesium.
- May Improve Heart Health.
- Can Lower Blood Sugar Levels.
- High in Fiber.

Raspberry Root

Good Source of Nutrients and Antioxidants.
Red raspberry leaves are rich in vitamins and minerals. They provide B vitamins,
vitamin C and several minerals, including potassium, magnesium, zinc,
phosphorus and iron. Adding nutrients and flavor to tea.

Red Clover Leaf

Red clover may be used for cancer prevention, indigestion, high cholesterol,
whooping cough, cough, asthma, bronchitis, and sexually transmitted diseases
(STDs). Some women use red clover for symptoms of menopause such as hot
flashes; for breast pain or tenderness (mastalgia); and for premenstrual syndrome
(PMS). Found in many herbal teas.

Rhodiola

Here are 7 possible health benefits of Rhodiola Rosea.

- Can Decrease Stress.
- Can Fight Fatigue.
- Could Help Reduce Symptoms of Depression.
- Improves Brain Function.
- Can Improve Exercise Performance.
- May Help Control Diabetes.
- May Have Anticancer Properties.

Rose Hips

Rosehips are the seed-filled red-orange pods that form at the base of the rose bloom. When boiled with water, they produce tea with a tangy, tart flavor and pinkish color. Notable for its high concentration of vitamin C, the herb is valued for its immune-strengthening properties (some consider it superior to most vitamin C supplements). Any tea with a berry or fruit flavor typically contains rosehips.

Rose Petals

May help in Removing Toxins: Rose tea may help prevent urinary tract infections due to its detox and diuretic properties. Boosts Immunity: To lose weight in a healthy way, it's essential for you to be free of illnesses first and rose tea may help you fight infections, due to the presence of vitamin C in it. Rose petals are a very rich source of vitamin A, C and E which can help hydrate and tighten the skin and reduce the appearance of wrinkles and dark circles. Roses contain anti-bacterial and anti-inflammatory properties, making this delicious herbal tea an ideal home cure for various skin conditions including, acne.

Rooibos (Green) Rooibos (Red) Rooibos

The Benefits of Rooibos Teas

- Improves blood pressure and circulation. Inflammation is a key player in the role of heart disease.
- Keeps hair strong and skin healthy. The benefits of rooibos tea go beyond just making a tea from it.
- May Aid in weight loss.
- May treats and help prevents diabetes.
- May help prevent some cancers.
- Boosts bone health.

Roasted Burdock Root

- Improving blood sugar and treating diabetes.
- Treating and preventing infections.
- 'Purifying' the blood.
- Diuretic.
- Antioxidant.
- Reducing inflammation.
- May help in treating or preventing cancer.

Rose Hips

May be helpful in any of the following:

- Immune Boosting. One of nature's richest sources of vitamin C, Rosehips have been used for centuries to combat infections such as coughs, colds, flu and respiratory conditions.
- Arthritis.
- Digestive Health.
- Weight Loss.

Rosemary

Here are 5 potential health benefits and uses of rosemary tea.

High in antioxidant, antimicrobial, and anti-inflammatory compounds.
May help lower your blood sugar.
May improve your mood and memory.
May support brain health.

May protect vision and eye health.

Sage

Here are 8 benefits and uses of sage tea.

- Rich in anti-inflammatory and antioxidant compounds.
- May promote healthy skin and wound healing.
- Helps promotes oral health.
- May have anticancer properties.
- May help to improves blood sugar control.
- May promote brain health and improve mood.
- May support women's health.
- May boost heart health.

Sarsaparilla

Sarsaparilla is used for treating psoriasis and other skin diseases, rheumatoid arthritis (RA), and kidney disease; for increasing urination to reduce fluid retention; and for increasing sweating. Sarsaparilla is also used along with conventional drugs for treating leprosy and for syphilis. May be mixed with other herbs for a great tasting refreshing tea.

Saw Palmetto

Saw palmetto is a species of palm used to produce a supplement that's packed with health benefits. Promising recent research shows that saw palmetto may help increase testosterone levels, improve prostate health, reduce inflammation, prevent hair loss, and enhance urinary tract function.

Schisandra

Schisandra Benefits
- Stress & Anxiety. Schisandra is likely that it is a powerful anti-anxiety herb, in addition to its ability to boost one's mood through lowering stress levels and enhancing mental performance.
- Longevity.
- Anti-Inflammatory.
- Skin Health.

Sencha Green

Potential benefits of sencha green tea include:

- Possible anti-cancer properties.
- May aid weight-loss.
- Useful with anti-aging properties.
- May help with prevention of neurodegenerative diseases.
- Help with anti-inflammatory properties.
- Help with lowering bad cholesterol.
- Useful anti-bacterial properties.
- Help prevention of some bacterial and virus infections.

Spearmint

8 Common Benefits of Spearmint Tea and Essential Oil

- Good for Digestive Upsets. Spearmint is commonly used to help relieve symptoms of indigestion, nausea, vomiting and gas.
- High in Antioxidants.
- May Aid Women with Hormone Imbalances.
- May Reduce Facial Hair in Women.
- May Improve Memory.
- Fights Bacterial Infections.
- May Lower Blood Sugar.
- May Help Reduce Stress.

Stevia Leaf

- Health Benefits. Substitute for Sugar
- Stevia May Help Control Blood Sugar and Insulin Levels.
- Stevia May Help Lower Blood Pressure.
- A Sweetener That's Good for Your Teeth.
  Fights Cavities.
  May Benefits Diabetes and Metabolic Syndrome.
  Helps Prevent Ear and Upper Respiratory Infections.

Stinging Nettles

 Here are 6 benefits of stinging nettle.
- Contains Many Nutrients. Stinging nettle's leaves and root provide a wide variety of nutrients, including (1):
- May Reduce Inflammation.
- May Treat Enlarged Prostate Symptoms.
- May Treat Hay Fever.
- May Lower Blood Pressure.
- May Aid Blood Sugar Control.

Thyme

Thyme essential oil, which is obtained from its leaves, is often used as a natural cough remedy. In one study, a combination of thyme and ivy leaves helped to alleviate coughing and other symptoms of acute bronchitis. Next time you're faced with a cough or sore throat, try drinking some thyme tea.

Turmeric Root

Drinking turmeric tea is believed to bring about several benefits, nine of which are described in more detail here. The newest rediscovered healing herb.

- Help Reduces arthritis symptoms.
- Help Boosts immune function.
- Helps reduce cardiovascular complications.
- Helps prevent and treat cancer.
- Helps manage irritable bowel syndrome or IBS.
- Prevents and treats Alzheimer's.

Valerian Root

Valerian tea is an herbal beverage made from the roots and underground stems of the valerian plant. Possible benefits of drinking the tea include improved sleep, decreased stress, menstrual symptom relief, and even a reduction of menopausal symptoms.

Yerba Mate

- Rich in Antioxidants and Nutrients.
- Can Boost Energy and Improve Mental Focus.
- May Enhance Physical Performance.
- May Protect Against Infections.
- May Help You Lose Weight and Belly Fat.
- May Boost Your Immune System.

Watermelon Rind

- May boost libido.
- Workout booster.
- Reduces blood pressure.
- Rich in fiber.
- Takeaway.

Watermelon Seed

Historically used as a diuretic for kidney and bladder cleansing, Watermelon Seed prepared from the cut seed as a tea is a simple home remedy that promotes urinary and cardiovascular health and may assist with diabetes and weight loss management.

Wheatgrass

- High in Nutrients and Antioxidants.
- May Reduce Cholesterol. Cholesterol is a waxy substance found throughout the body.
- Could Help Kill Cancer Cells.
- May Aid in Blood Sugar Regulation.
- May Alleviate Inflammation.
- Could Help Promote Weight Loss.
- Easy to Add to Your Teas. Drink as a hot or cold beverage.

Wild Yam

Diosgenin or wild yam is often promoted as a "natural alterative" to estrogen therapy, so you will see it used for estrogen replacement therapy, vaginal dryness in older women, PMS (premenstrual syndrome), menstrual cramps, weak bones (osteoporosis), increasing energy and sexual drive in men and women, and breast.

Brief description of Tonics:

A **tonic** is a medicine that makes you feel stronger, healthier, and less tired. In short, **tonics** are herbal in nature and provide nutritional support to an area of the body. The use of these herbs in their not-standardized-form provides key support for the health and function of that part of your body. ... Using **tonic** herbs helps bring balance to our body.

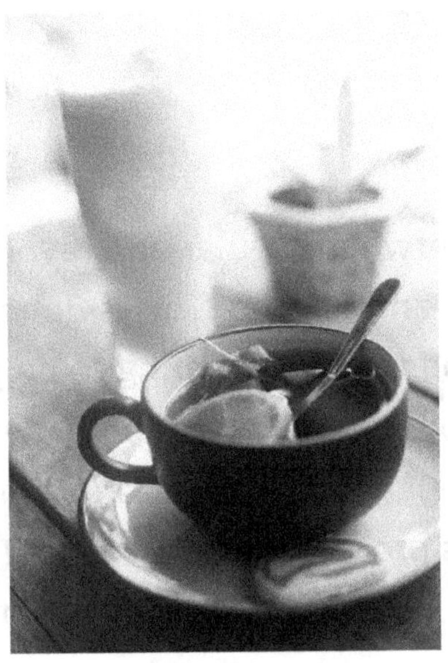

<u>Tonic Tea</u>- To strengthen your whole body for vital energy.

<u>Eastern Tonics</u>- Ginseng Root, Dong Quai Root

<u>Western Tonics</u>- Sage Leaves, whole plant of Rosemary

<u>South American Tonics</u>- Suma Root, Yerba Mate Leaves

The Difference Between Regular and Raw Honey

When you see recipes with honey, you may be wondering why just grabbing a plastic bear full of the stuff won't work as well. You may be wondering what the difference is and how to make sure you are choosing the right honey for the job. You may also be wondering how to find the right raw honey and labeling differences to look for. Here are some of the differences to look for and why you need to look for them.

Pasteurization

One of the key differences between regular and raw honey is how it is processed. Regular honey is pasteurized and filtered. This is done to prevent fermentation of the honey while it is sitting on the shelf waiting to be purchased or while it travels through different climates to the selling location. One way to tell if the honey you are buying has been put through this process is to simply look at it. If it is clear then it has gone through this process. Real raw honey has a milky like color and has small grains. These grains melt in hot water or hot liquid.

Check the Vitamins

One easy way to see if the raw honey you are buying is truly raw is to check the nutrition label. The nutrition label will list what vitamins and nutrients, along with the percentages of each, are in the honey. If you don't see any, or if certain ones like Vitamin B, aren't listed then you know it isn't raw. Raw honey contains Vitamins A, C, D, E and B-complex. Also look for something called amylase. This is an enzyme you will only find in raw honey. This helps with digestion and with stomach issues.

Antibacterial and Soothing

You can also test the honey by using it on sore throats and wounds. If it doesn't work, or only helps for a few minutes, then you know it isn't raw. Overall, raw honey will work for several hours on a sore throat and will help with wound healing. It is evident if it is working or just putting a sugary substance on the infected area.

By keeping these three differences in mind, and what to look for, you can make the right choice between regular and raw honey. You can also begin using raw honey for the benefits to your health and not just the taste.

Herbal Teas That Taste Great with Honey

If you are a tea drinker, you may be wondering what teas you can easily add honey too without making them too sweet. Though there are the traditional black teas, there are other teas that taste great with honey. Here are a few of those teas and how you can easily make them yourself or how to make them without having them turn out too sweet.

Fruit Based Teas

Most fruit based herbal teas taste great with honey. You can make these yourself easily by just using citrus based fruits or dried fruits like strawberries. Boil water add the fruits, and then add some raw honey. You can drain it if necessary or eat the fruit. You can also buy fruit loose leaf tea blends that are easy to mix with honey and easy to store. Though you can buy pre-bagged fruit teas, finding a loose-leaf option or making your own is best because it gives you the whole fruits and not just the powdered processed versions. This means you are getting more of the benefits.

Chamomile

Chamomile is known for its calming effects, but sometimes the taste may not be ideal. In fact, if you have an upset stomach or if you are giving it to a teenager, the taste may be off putting. If that is the case, then adding honey may be ideal. You will not only get the benefits of the chamomile, but you will also gain the digestive benefits of the honey which can calm your body and help soothe your stomach. This can help you sleep better and make the tea palatable.

Green Tea

If you are on a weight loss journey, then you probably already use green tea in your daily routine. Even if you use it once a week or more you may know that the taste can be a bit bitter. This is especially true if you are using green tea that is a loose leaf or organic option instead of pre-bagged cheaper options. You may be using sugar to help offset this taste, but even then it doesn't do much to mask the bitterness. What can help and can boost the weight loss properties of your green tea, is to add raw honey. Major brands have already proven how well honey works with green tea in iced tea formulas, and the same can be said for hot tea as well.

If you are concerned with adding honey to your tea when you are on the go, consider carrying raw honey sticks with you. They are easy to carry, easy to store, and can easily be added to any of the tea you order while out. You can also get flavored raw honey sticks that as well can add cinnamon or other flavors.

Juice Recipes with Raw Honey

If you have been juicing, then you may already have your juicing routine down. In fact, most people who juice stick to one or two recipes that work well for them. If this sounds like you, but your juicing is starting to get a bit old and you want to boost it, then you may be wondering the best way to make a change that helps but isn't dramatic. One way you can do this is to add raw honey to your juicing. Here are a few recipes that you can try and see how they work for you.

Energy Boosting Juice with Raw Honey

Raw honey is known as a natural energy boosting agent. This is even better if you mix it with other energy boosting superfoods in a morning juice. This juice can be made easily with cucumbers, apple, and raw honey. Simply juice down the apple and cucumber like you would normally do. Strain the juice if necessary and add raw honey. This gives you a hydration boost with the cucumbers being over 90 percent water. It also gives you the energy from the honey and the vitamins and minerals from the apples. It is easy, and easy to find all the ingredients year-round. You can even grow cucumbers indoors if you want.

Digestive Boosting Juice with Raw Honey

Orange, aloe vera, and spinach can make a powerful digestive juice. It can help flush your system and keep it regular. It can also get you back to a regular digestive tract depending on your needs. The problem with this juice is that some people can taste too much of the spinach or feel like the aloe vera makes the drink to dilute. If this is the case, you can add raw honey to the juice. It will offer more digestive boosters and help flavor the drink to cover the spinach or the dilution that you may taste on the first try.

Immune Boosting Juice with Raw Honey

Immune boosting juices are popular during cold and flu season or when you start or change your diet routine. For that reason, most people want the most potent immune boosting juice they can find. One of the easiest juices is carrot, apple, and orange. All three of these have immune boosting properties but adding raw honey to the mix can give it even more. You can find all the ingredients year-round and all are inexpensive.

These three juice recipes are based on very common and easy to make juices. Regardless of where you are located, you should be able to find these ingredients year-round and adjust the recipes accordingly to your tastes.

Raw Honey vs Bee Pollen

When you start buying supplements, you may be buying them based on what you know of them. This is fine, until you have a cabinet full of supplements and you haven't cross referenced them to see what they do and if you are overlapping some of the supplements you are taking. One of the confusing supplement options is bee pollen. If you are already using raw honey, then you may want to know what benefit bee pollen will have. Here is what you should know about the differences between each.

Fatigue Reduction

One of the key points to note between raw honey and bee pollen is what it can do for fatigue levels. If you suffer from chronic fatigue issues then you may want to take bee pollen over raw honey. Yes, raw honey does help with energy boosting, but it does not help with long term fatigue issues and the root causes of those issues. So, the difference in this area is that raw honey is a quick fix to energy boosting like boosting energy in the afternoon when you start to feel tired or before a workout. Bee pollen is more of a long-term option that can be taken daily for CFS issues.

Allergy Reduction

Raw honey is something you can use in your daily routine to help reduce allergy symptoms. This does help during allergy seasons to boost your immune system and to boost your reduction to allergy causing agents like pollen. However, if you have long term issues then you may find bee pollen is an ideal option. Just like with fatigue issues, bee pollen helps with long term effects instead of instant or relatively instant effects of raw honey. Most people that use honey for allergy issues do use both in some mixture throughout the day.

Production

One of the key things to remember about the difference between raw honey and bee pollen is how it is produced. Raw honey is produced over time by bees. Bee pollen is the flower pollen that bees carry with them during the pollination process. Bee pollen is the pollen that creates the honey while the honey is the end product of the pollination process.

By keeping these three key points in mind, you can make the better choice on which one you want to take and how you want to mix it into your daily routine. You may find that taking both works, or that taking one or the other at different parts of the year works best.

If you are interested in a new kind of honey called Shungite Honey please visit this website for more information: www.mysticalwears.net

Honey Water 101

Honey water is a drink that you may have heard of, but you may know very little to nothing about. The truth is honey water is easy to make, easy to mix, and offers several benefits especially for those people on a weight loss journey. If you are thinking of using honey water, or at least trying it, in your diet then consider these key points about the drink and how to use it properly.

Making Honey Water

Making honey water is very easy. The key thing to remember is the amount of honey you start with and that adding to that amount is okay, after you taste it. You don't want the water too sweet. It should not be like drinking sugar water. Your first step is to boil water as if you are making tea. Remove the water from the heat and add one to two tablespoons of honey. If you are measuring this in grams, it should be between 15 and 30 grams. Adjust this to taste.

When to Take it and How

You can drink the water first thing in the morning or right after your coffee or tea. You can also drink it at other times during the day. Some people using it for weight loss tend to drink it twice a day, once in the morning and once in the evening before bed. The key to using honey water is to drink it hot or at the very least warm. You need to drink it like a tea. Now, you may be wondering if you can add things to your honey water. You can. You can add apple cider vinegar to help with cleansing, orange to give a boost of Vitamin C for your immune system, or even lemon. Ginger is also an additive than can help boost your immune system.

Increasing Weight Loss

Weight loss assistance is one reason that many people use honey water in their daily routine. It can help with digestive issues that may prevent or pose an obstacle to weight loss. The water flushes the system, helps with constipation, and helps keep you regular so you aren't holding onto extra weight or bloat. It can also help reduce cravings for sugar which is an issue for many people on their weight loss journey. Energy during weight loss can also be an issue and raw honey does offer natural energy boosting properties.

This is just the basic information regarding honey water. Keep in mind, by starting to use this water daily you will notice a difference in your body. Make sure to note those differences and adjust the honey water accordingly.

How to Add More Raw Honey to Your Diet

You know that there are health benefits to raw honey, but you may not know the best ways to add it to your diet. In fact, you may be concerned about adding it to certain foods because it may make them overly sweet. The truth is, there are three very easy ways to add raw honey to your diet and get the benefits that you need.

Adding to Your Morning Tea

Instead of adding sugar to your tea, grab the raw honey instead. The trick to this is, if you use a coffeehouse or coffee chain to get your morning coffee, you will want to have your own raw honey on hand instead of theirs. This is because most coffee shops do not store raw honey and use commercial processed honey instead.

Before you think this may be tougher than you think, consider that most health food stores do sell raw honey in straw form. You can pack a few straws and take them with you in your purse or bag. The honey sticks equal about one teaspoon of raw honey and can easily be added after you order your coffee.

Use Instead of Syrup

If you have pancakes or waffles in the morning, or if you add syrup or sugar to your oatmeal, consider using raw honey instead. You do not need as much of it to get the sweet flavor you are looking for. It also will give you the benefits you need throughout the day including a burst of energy.

Add to Energy Bars

One of the easiest ways to add raw honey to your diet is to make your own energy bars and use a daily serving of honey in each bar. This will make it easy for you to know how much you are getting in a serving. It will also replace the sugars that you would normally use in the energy bars. Make sure you are making a superfood bar to increase the benefits. You can have this energy bar at lunch, for a snack, or as part of a dessert for your lunch.

These are the three easiest ways to add raw honey to your diet. Try these and expand the uses out to other foods and other points in your day. You may be surprised how easy it is to add it into your daily routine.

How to Use Honey for Weight Loss

Weight loss journeys are all different. Everyone has a different plan, a different goal, and different obstacles in their lives. One of the things that everyone can benefit from on their weight loss journey is honey. Specifically, the benefits found in raw honey. If you are starting a weight loss journey, here are a few of the ways you can use it to help with that weight loss.

Honey Water

Drinking honey water in the morning and at night can help you boost your energy and your immune system. Having a healthy immune system is important during your weight loss journey. As you change the foods you eat and your lifestyle, you will notice that your energy level may drop and that you are having issues with getting sick. Your body is adapting and trying to adapt to your new routine, and this can make it switch gears a little too quickly. Honey water helps with that by delivering the raw nutrients of raw honey directly to your system in an easy to use method.

Digestive Assistance

Your digestion during weight loss is equally as important as all the other focuses on your journey. As you change your diet and your routine, you will notice an increase in your bowels. Unfortunately, this may not last and you may start having issues with constipation due to the change in foods and increase in supplements or energy bars. If this is the case you will need digestive assistance to keep things regular and to make sure that you aren't bloated or retaining water.

Sugar Replacement

One of the foods that will prevent you from dropping the weight you want and from moving forward in your weight loss journey is sugar. Sugar can be in most of the foods you eat and can take a toll even when you think it isn't. For example, you may think that just having sugar in your coffee is fine, but that does add up. Instead switch to honey and use it as a sugar replacement. Try to stick to raw honey which has less of a processed sugar taste and gives you the nutrients you need.

By putting these three weight loss methods into action, where raw honey is concerned, you will start to notice that it is easier to drop the weight and to keep your sugar intake to a minimum. You will also notice less cravings which can help during tougher points of the weight loss journey.

Health Benefits of Raw Honey

Raw honey is something you see in many DIY recipes and health food recipes. Unfortunately, most of these recipes do not tell you why the honey is added or the benefits it will have to your body as a whole. This may leave you wondering why you should add it, why you should use specifically raw honey, and what benefits it is going to give to your body. Here are a few of the answers that may help you make the choice for raw honey in the future.

All-In-One

One of the leading benefits of raw honey is that is an all-in-one remedy that can replace several of your current supplements. For example, if you are taking supplements for anti-inflammatory or for digestive issues and antioxidants than consider chunking them in the bin and going with just raw honey. Raw honey is antibacterial, antifungal, anti-inflammatory, and is loaded with antioxidants. It even helps with digestive issues that range from constipation to upset stomachs and ulcers.

Reduction of Allergies

Allergies are an issue for many people, and some have them more severe than others. If you are having to load up on allergy medicine everyday just to get through your day without a headache, or if you are tired of being tired from the same medicine, then raw honey may be ideal. You can use honey water daily, and it will start to have lasting effects within a few days to a few weeks. This does not help on its own. You will need to make sure that you take additional steps, such as cleaning your home and vacuuming or using hepa filters throughout your home to help reduce the allergy causing agents as well.

Natural Energy

Natural energy is one of the key reasons that many people have turned to raw honey in their diet and especially in their weight loss journey's. You can take just a few spoonsful of raw honey a day or add it to your coffee in the morning. You'll find after a few tries of this that you won't need the costly and dangerous energy drinks you've been taking when your afternoon crash hits. You will also see an increase in energy before your workouts as well.

These benefits are the three main benefits that raw honey can offer you. Remember, raw honey is the most pure and organic form you can buy. If the honey is not raw it may be cut with processed sugars and other preservatives that take away from the health benefits. One way to check for raw honey is either looking on the label or buying honey that has a piece of the honeycomb in it.

The Truth About Detox Teas

There is a long history of detox practices that litters the history of humanity. This idea is nothing new… there has been leeches and bloodletting, fasting and enemas, saunas and sweat lodges, herbs and teas. Many of these practices were used as medical treatments right until the 20th century. Teas have appeared as a popular detox method now, too. You'll have likely seen a variety of detox teas being pushed by celebrity influencers on social media. So, it's important that we address detox teas.

First, like most dietary supplements, there is no FDA regulation that covers detox teas. Some of these teas have been discovered to contain dangerous chemicals and drugs that don't appear on the packaging's ingredients list. So, you may have looked at the ingredients and recognized the ingredients, all of which are normal, but some of them may include other ingredients. You should never use any detox product before consulting your physician.

The reason that people look to detox teas is that we generally view teas as being a healthy drink. It's something that is consumed widely, and many herbal teas have additional health benefits. For example, green tea is viewed as healthy because it helps burn fat while you exercise.

What Detox Teas Do

There are no studies that prove detox tea will help you lose weight. In fact, if you look at the instructions that accompany many detox teas, they tell you to exercise, diet, and cleanse. They suggest that you eat very little or eat healthily. Often, the companies that push detox teas are telling you to exercise vigorously.

So, when you combine vigorous exercise with healthy (or little) eating, you are bound to lose weight. Ultimately, you will be losing weight because of that hard work, not because of some detox tea. Your change in lifestyle will encourage your liver and kidneys to do their natural detoxification job.

There is another risk of detox tea. They're often high in caffeine. Most teas contain caffeine. When you have a high level of caffeine present, however, it acts as a diuretic. This will cause you to lose water weight, but it isn't real weight loss. Additionally, this laxative effect that detox teas have will speed up the digestion process. Your abdomen will look flatter and you will feel slimmer. This isn't lasting weight loss. What it can do is seriously dehydrate you, which will put your health at risk.

Side Effects of Detox Teas

There are detox teas which are completely harmless, they are merely an assortment of tea leaves. However, there are those that contain powerful and dangerous ingredients like medications, ephedra, Senna, laxatives, and high levels of caffeine. The purpose of these ingredients is to provide you with energy and to create weight loss through frequent restroom visits. You aren't purging toxins this way; you're simply losing water weight.

The ingredients designed to speed you up can create dangerous issues such as seizures, heart attacks, strokes, and even death.

Typical side effects include:

• Diarrhea – detox teas often feature laxatives. A laxative is normally safe to use when you follow the instructions. However, when you are consuming this tea regularly, it can cause diarrhea and completely dehydrate you. It will also upset normal digestion when you use them for an extended period. You may reach a point where you are reliant on them just to have a normal bowel movement.

• Cramps – a common side effect of detox tea, cramp, as well as gas, bloating, and stomach pains. The reason for this is the stress that caffeine and laxatives have on your digestive system.

• Electrolyte Imbalance – the more you visit the bathroom, the more dehydrated you will become which can result in a loss of electrolytes which your muscles require to function.

Additionally, excess caffeine intake can cause irritation, agitation, anxiety, nervousness, headaches, restlessness, an increase in heart rate, and disruption to sleep. You don't need to drink detox tea in order to follow a detox diet. Water is a safer and more powerful detox solution.

Natural Herbs to Fight Fatigue

If you have been feeling exhausted lately, to the point where it doesn't feel like just being tired or lack of sleep, but overwhelming fatigue, it is time to do something about it.

There are many causes of fatigue, as well as many ways to treat it. Sometimes it is a matter of treating the cause of your fatigue, but in other cases, you just need to experiment with a few different remedies until you figure out what works best for you.

The following information is going to guide you through some natural remedies for fatigue, particularly by using medicinal herbs. These herbs provide a lot of health benefits for you, so while they can help with your fatigue, they will also help with other ailments at the same time.

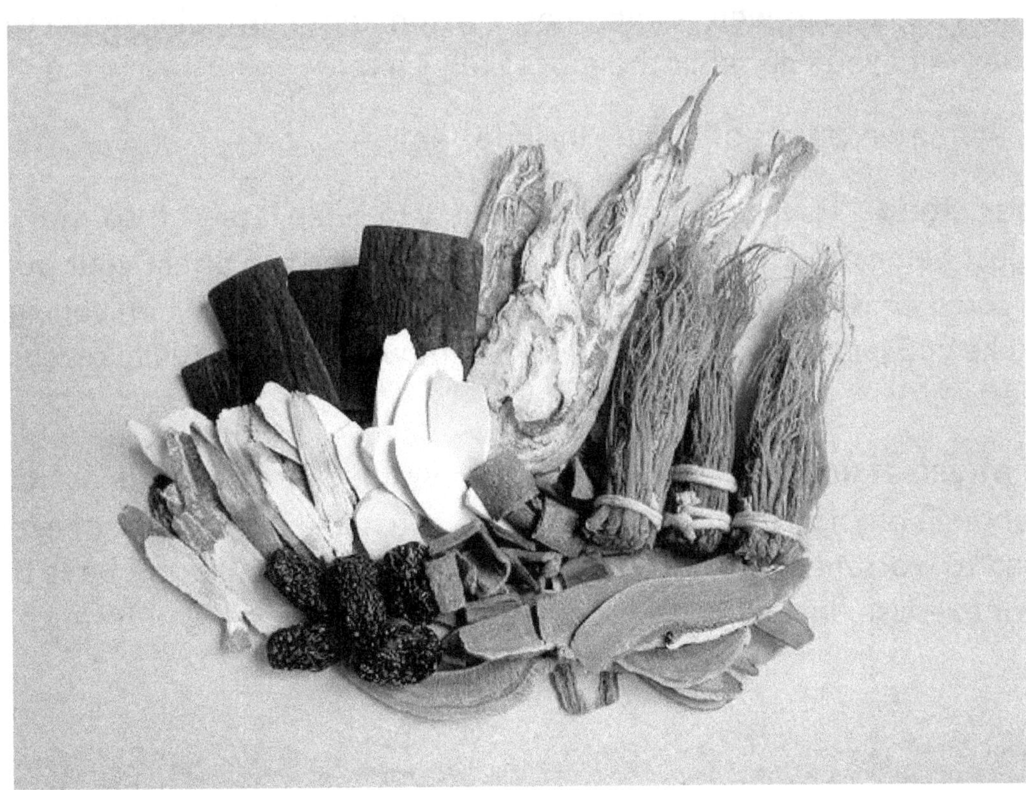

1. Common Causes of Fatigue

There are two basic types of fatigue – acute and chronic. Acute fatigue tends to be short-term and easier to treat and is most associated with lifestyle choices like diet and lack of exercise. Then there is chronic fatigue, which can also be from lifestyle stressors, but is also associated with medical conditions. Chronic fatigue may go away temporarily but is more of a long-term struggle.

In both cases, the fatigue might be from any number of causes, and can be caused by more than one thing at a time. Before you look at the natural herbs and other natural remedies that will help with your fatigue, it helps to understand what might be causing it.

Most Common Causes of Fatigue

First, if you have been struggling with fatigue for a while, you should look at the most common culprits first. Some of these might sound familiar to you, but don't rule out other causes as well. Sometimes, it just means narrowing down the possibilities until you figure out the most likely factor.

The most common causes of fatigue include:

Improper sleep – Have you been struggling with sleep lately? If so, you might go from just being tired to having fatigue, where it starts to affect your quality of life. This could be issues with falling asleep, staying asleep, or when you wake up, you feel like you just tossed and turned all night without ever really reaching a deep sleep.

Lack of physical activity – Another very common cause of fatigue is not getting enough physical activity. This can be a catch 22 because lack of exercise might lead to worsened fatigue, but you are so tired that you don't have the energy for exercise. Just adding a little at a time can make a big difference.

Poor diet – Your diet can also affect your sleep and cause fatigue for various reasons. This might include an unhealthy diet and not getting enough nutrients, eating too little and facing malnutrition, or eating at times when it affects your sleep, such as late at night immediately before bedtime.

Anemia – Among the physical conditions that can lead to fatigue, anemia is one of the most common ones. You might be susceptible to anemia, or it may be caused by not having enough iron in your diet.

Fatigue disorder – Another condition is a fatigue disorder, which is one of the more common causes of chronic fatigue. This will require help from your doctor.

Mental issues – Don't forget about your mental health, as things like stress, anxiety, depression, and other mental health conditions can greatly affect your energy levels and sleep patterns. This in turn can cause some major chronic fatigue.

Possible Lifestyle Causes

In addition to diet and exercise, there are some other lifestyle factors to consider when it comes to why you are struggling with fatigue. For example, if you travel a lot, you might be suffering from something called jet lag disorder. This has to do with your lifestyle and is something you will need to work on in order to get proper sleep.

Another possibility is that you are taking medications that are causing more fatigue, even if you think they are helping, such as too many antihistamines or medication meant to cause drowsiness to help you sleep at night.

You should also limit your use of drugs and alcohol, as they can also lead to fatigue and sleep disturbances.

Medical Conditions Causing Fatigue

If you have fatigue that is more chronic, it is a good time to talk to your doctor. They will run some tests and rule out any possible medical causes for the fatigue. Here is a list of some of the more common conditions, but it is by no means a complete list:

Inflammatory bowel disease
acute liver failure
Chronic kidney disease
Diabetes
Fibromyalgia
Infection or inflammation
Chronic obstructive pulmonary disease
Sleep apnea
Recent traumatic injury
Thyroid issues

As you can see, fatigue is very complex. There is a long list of possible causes, so it is a good idea to start writing down when you experience fatigue, how long it lasts, and what was going on before it occurred.

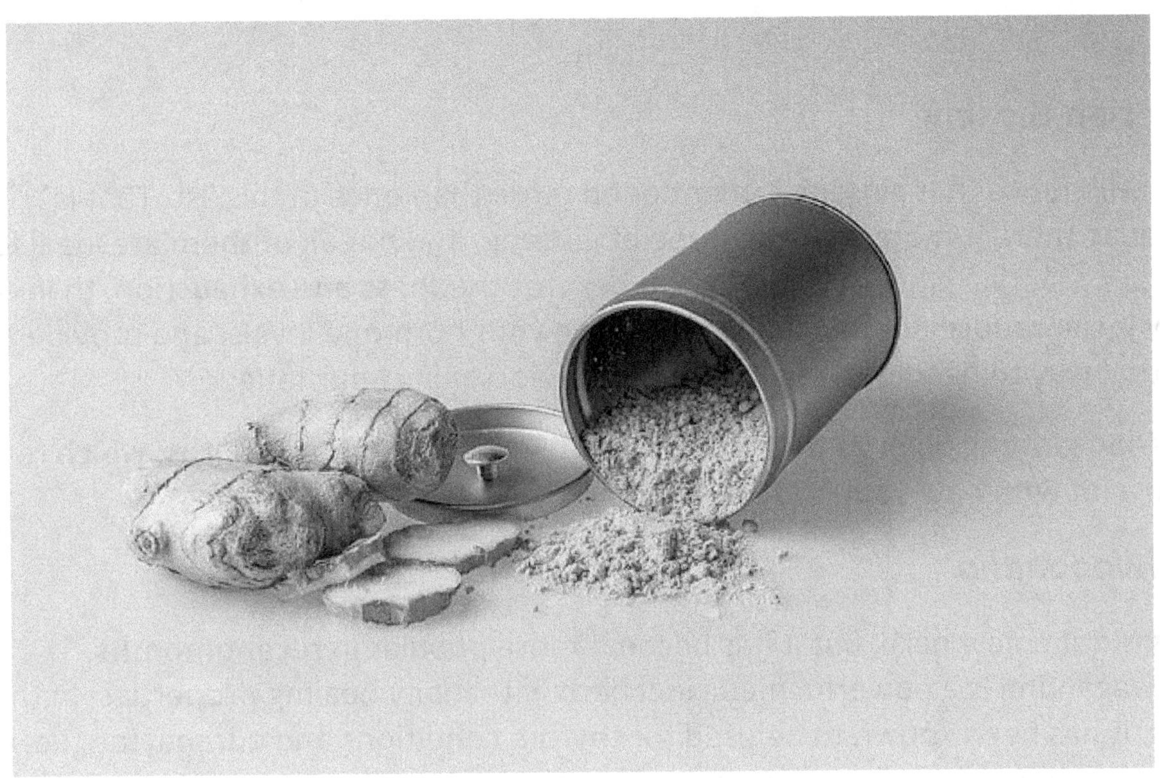

2. Herbs That Fight Fatigue

While there are many natural remedies for fatigue – many of which will be covered in a later section – medicinal herbs are a great place to start. They are easy to use, convenient and affordable, and you can get them just about anywhere. You can buy the dried or fresh herbs, or even grow them right in your own backyard.

Here are some of the top herbs that can help with your fatigue.

Licorice Root

This is one of the most popular herbs to be used for fatigue. Licorice root helps in a variety of ways, first be helping to repair your adrenals if they have been damaged, which can happen by some of the medical conditions that cause fatigue. Licorice root can also be helpful be reducing your cravings your sugar, which might cause a sugar crash and make your fatigue worse.

Additionally, licorice root has been shown to help reduce fatigue thanks to increasing the cortisol levels in your body. These are hormones that help you to experience more energy.

Siberian Ginseng

You will notice that ginseng is mentioned more than once in this list. That is because there is more than one type of ginseng, and not all of them are ideal for fatigue. Siberian ginseng is one of the best for tiredness and exhaustion, thanks to how it can reduce adrenal fatigue, improve your hormone levels, and provide a natural way to handle stress that might be worsening your fatigue.

Siberian ginseng belongs to a group of herbs called adaptogen herbs, which really help a lot with how your body can handle stress.

Ashwagandha

This is not a new herb, but it has become more popular in recent months. Ashwagandha is a powerful medicinal herb with many healing properties. In the past, it has been known to be used for thyroid conditions and adrenal fatigue, but of which you already know can lead to chronic fatigue if not treated properly.

Like many other healing herbs on this list, ashwagandha also helps to balance out your hormone levels. Another great way to increase your energy or reduce fatigue.

Maca

You might have heard of maca or maca root, and that is because it has become a well-known medicinal herb. Maca is a type of plant like cruciferous vegetables. These plants provide a natural energy like what you would get if you had caffeine, but without feeling the side effects like jitters.

When you have maca on a routine basis instead of caffeine, you are increasing your energy more naturally without all those nasty side effects. You don't get a sugar crash or nervous shakes that keep you from being productive. The bonus is that maca also has many other natural healing abilities, so you are helping with other bodily functions in addition to helping with your fatigue.

Ephedra

If this herb sounds familiar, it is because it used to be used in some form to create stimulating medications, however it should only be used in its natural form. Ephedra is a type of herbal medicine that helps to stave off fatigue while increasing your energy. However, it has some side effects that can be unwelcome, so it is best to consult an herbalist when using this one.

Asian Ginseng

As we mentioned, there is more than one variety of ginseng that can help with fatigue, including Asian ginseng. You might also see this labeled as panax ginseng. Asian ginseng is another popular Chinese medicinal herb that will help to improve functions in your body in order to increase your energy levels. As another adaptogen herb, this is vital to helping to control your chronic fatigue, while helping with your mental health and heart health at the same time.

Ginkgo Biloba

This is yet another healing herb that is familiar and great for fatigue. Ginkgo biloba is one of the oldest trees on Earth, so you can imagine how many different ailments it has helped with. This is a prescription medication in some countries, including Germany.

Ginkgo biloba is wonderful for oxidative stress, which is how it improves your adrenals and helps to fight fatigue naturally. It can also help to protect your liver and brain from free radicals in your body.

Sea Kelp

While not always known as an herb, sea kelp can also be great for your fatigue. The main purpose of sea kelp for fatigue is helping to treat your thyroid condition. It can help with low thyroid function and regulate your thyroid hormone levels, which helps to increase your energy naturally.

Gotu Kola

Moving on to the next herb is gotu kola. If you have ever researched Ayurvedic medicine for natural healing, then you might have come across this one. It grows in the Himalayas and is often used in ancient medicine. Gotu kola works like other healing herbs in that it helps to increase stamina and increase your energy.

Reishi Mushroom

A different type of herb is the reishi mushroom, which is found most often in Chinese herbal medicine. Reishi mushroom can be used in a tonic to help with your fatigue and increase your energy, while also helping to boost your immune system. It is also great for stress, which as you know can make your fatigue worse.

Stinging Nettle

When it comes to herbs, there are many different varieties that grow all over the world. Stinging nettle is one of those that tends to stick with you because of its name, and because of how many healing properties it contains.

This herb is used for a wide range of medicinal purposes, from helping to increase your energy, to providing a lot of essential vitamins and minerals for your physical and mental health. The great thing about stinging nettle is that it helps to improve your energy and stamina if you have fatigue, without all the negative side effects.

Ginger Root

Another adaptogen herb that is healing and easy to find is ginger root. This is like the ginger you use in cooking, but you are going to use it as a medicinal herb. Ginger has a long list of healing powers as you probably already know, from helping with digestive to providing a natural way of reducing pain and discomfort.

It is also wonderful if you have fatigue! It helps with adrenal fatigue like how ginseng and ginkgo biloba do. In addition to this, ginger root can regulate cortisol levels in your body and help to reduce your stress levels.

St. John's Wort

Last up is St. John's Worth, which you might have used as a natural remedy for depression or sleep issues. St. john's worth is easy to find at any drug store, not just the ones that carry natural herbal medicines. You can find it in many forms, from a pill you swallow, to powder and extract forms.

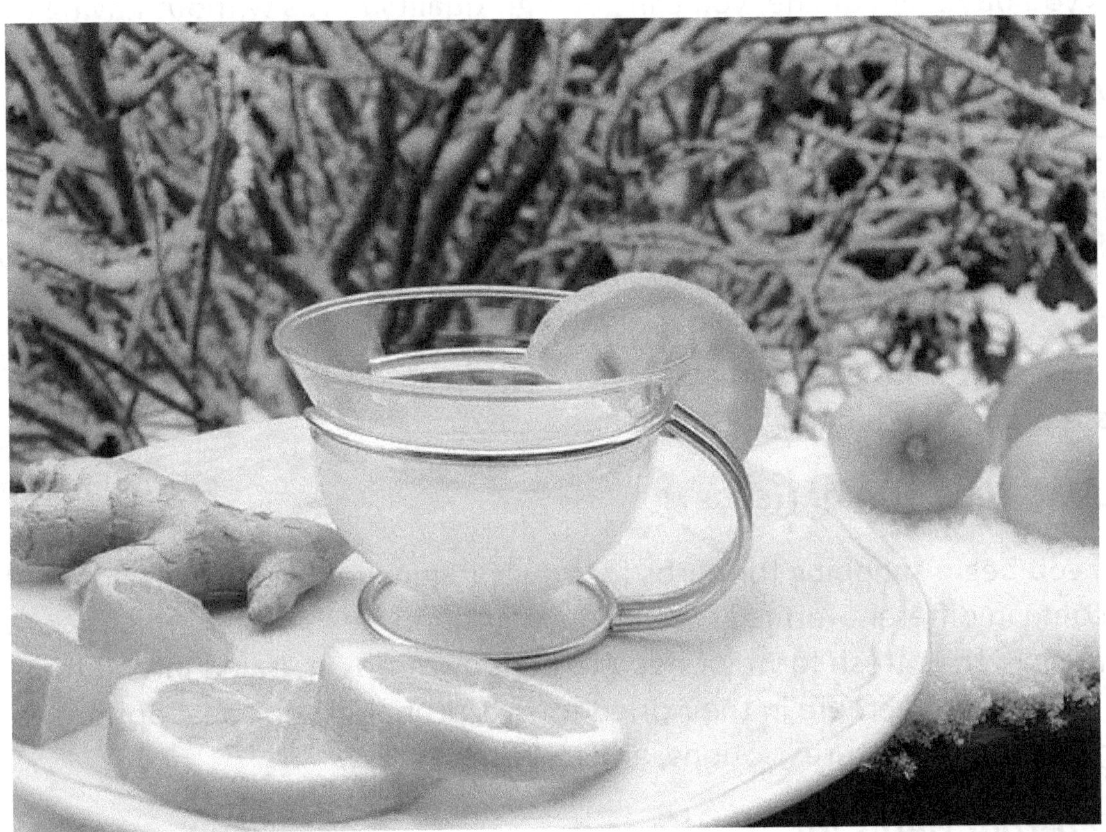

3. Tips for Using Herbs

The first step to fighting fatigue naturally is of course to learn the causes of your fatigue and select which herbs you want to use. Once you do that, there are a few things to understand, including how best to use the herbs.

Here are some tips for using your medicinal and healing herbs, not just for fatigue, but other uses as well.

Where to Buy the Herbs

You have a wide range of options when it comes to choosing the herbs, whether you grow them at home or decide to purchase them. If you have never purchased herbs before, then your two main options are in person or online.

When you buy them online, you can get high-quality herbs without having to drive to different stores in your area. This is especially useful if you don't have many markets or herbal shops in your area.

In person, there are even more options available to you. You can try a health food store if your regular supermarket does not supply the herbs you need. Another option is to go to a specialty herbal store or see a local herbalist to see if they have what you need.

You can also try farmer's markets, which often provide some homegrown herbs that are organic and the highest quality.

Selecting the Form of Herbs

When you begin shopping for herbs for your fatigue, you will quickly notice that they come in different forms as well. You might find fresh herbs, which you would either use in their fresh form, or need to dry on your own. If you intend to use dried herbs, getting them in their dried form is probably your best option. You can also get herbs as tinctures, lotions, and salves.

Testing Your Herbs for Reactions

Before you start using herbs to fight fatigue, you should test them by using a small amount one at a time. Don't just make a tea with 4 different healing herbs and hope for the best. You might have a bad reaction to one and won't know which one it is.

Decide how you are going to use the herbs for fatigue, then choose just one herb at a time, in a small amount. Consult a doctor immediately if you show signs of an allergic reaction, such as with swelling, redness, itching, or trouble breathing.

The last thing you should know about using herbs for fatigue is that there are a few different ways to use them. Here are some excellent ways to get more energy with your medicinal herbs:

Add them to a bath – This is a wonderful way to improve your adrenals, reduce stress, and help improve your fatigue at the same time. If your fatigue is related to being stressed or having adrenal fatigue, a hot bath with dried herbs is a wonderful way to use them.

Make a tea in the morning – For more energy in the morning when you likely experience a lot of fatigue, try making a cup of tea with your chosen herbs or herb blends. Tea with ginger, gingko biloba, or ginseng is a great option.

Infuse different oils – Don't forget about herb-infused oils! These can be made to add to food and drinks, making it easy to treat your fatigue and increase energy at the same time.

Put them on your skin directly – In some cases, you want to get the herbs into your skin instead of other methods. This is when you might make a poultice or salve. This not only helps with your fatigue but can help you to heal skin irritations as well.

4. Other Natural Remedies for Fatigue

While these medicinal herbs offer a great place for you to start managing your chronic fatigue, there are also some other natural remedies and lifestyle changes that can be very useful. It is good to try different things until you figure out what works best for you.

Stay Active

One good way to fight fatigue in a more natural way is to stay active. This might seem counter intuitive but being more active won't make you more tired, at least not in the way you think. Exercise gives you a good amount of energy during the waking hours, but then when it is time to wind down and get ready for bed, you will sleep much more soundly.

Pick any type of physical activity you like in order to get more exercise for energy but think about some that have other health benefits as well, like yoga. Yoga can really center you, help you with breathing exercises, reduce stress, and heal both your body and your mind.

Eat More Superfoods

Nutrition can also make a drastic difference in how well you are dealing with your fatigue, whether acute or chronic. Eating too many simple carbohydrates can cause your fatigue to be worsened, especially with sugar crashes in the afternoon. Try switching to a more balanced diet with lots of fresh fruits and veggies, nuts and seeds, lean protein, and healthy fats. Some good superfoods for energy include:

Bananas
Yogurt
Leafy greens
Nuts and seeds
Watermelon
Oatmeal
Green tea
Dark chocolate

Take Magnesium

Some supplements are better than others, but one of the best ones for fighting fatigue is magnesium. You can get this naturally in the foods you eat if you don't want to take another supplement in the morning. Magnesium is found in foods like whole grains, nuts, fish, and bananas.

Alchemy Tea Recipe Sample:

Lemon Honey Zinger (Green Tea)

* 1 (2 inch) piece lemon zest, cut into thin slivers
* 2 teaspoons green tea powder or two tea bags
* 1 3/4 cup hot water
* 1/4 cup freshly squeezed grapefruit juice
* 3 tablespoons freshly squeezed lemon juice
* 1 teaspoon honey
* May be served hot or cold. Mix all ingrediencies together let step in boiling water for 4 to 5 minutes. Place lemon slices in tea after it has steeped. Either drink hot or refrigerate and served cold. Makes 2 Cups.

Above is a sample of a Tea that I produced many years ago. I will have more recipes in the future books. Please keep track and add your comments on the website www.TheSpiritedAlchemy.com   You can also download a journal to keep track of your own recipes and results.

If you are looking for loose Healthy Healing Teas, here is a list of my Teas available to order online: Inquire about the ingrediencies I use.

Body Balance: **Diabetes-Cholesterol, Calorie Burner Support**

Heavenly Dreams: Relaxation and Sleep

Holy Harmony: Anti-depression, Mood balance

Holy Healing Joint Ease: Joints and arthritis

Spirited Stress Relief: Negative Stress Relief

Super Immunity Boost: Super Immunity

Available to Purchase on websites listed:

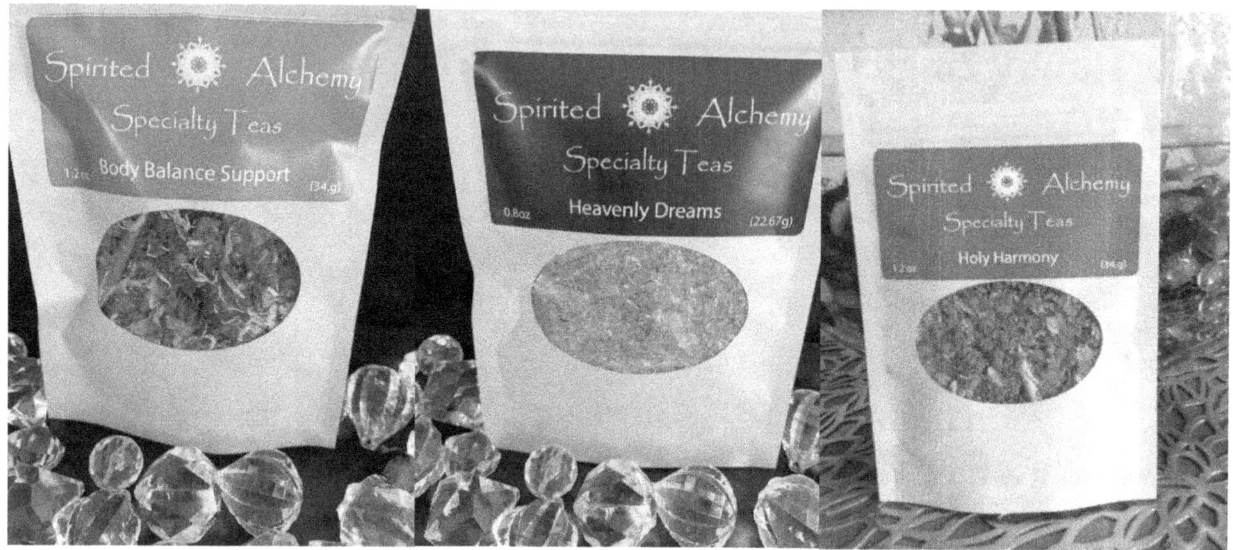

Body Balance Support **Heavenly Dreams** **Holy Harmony**

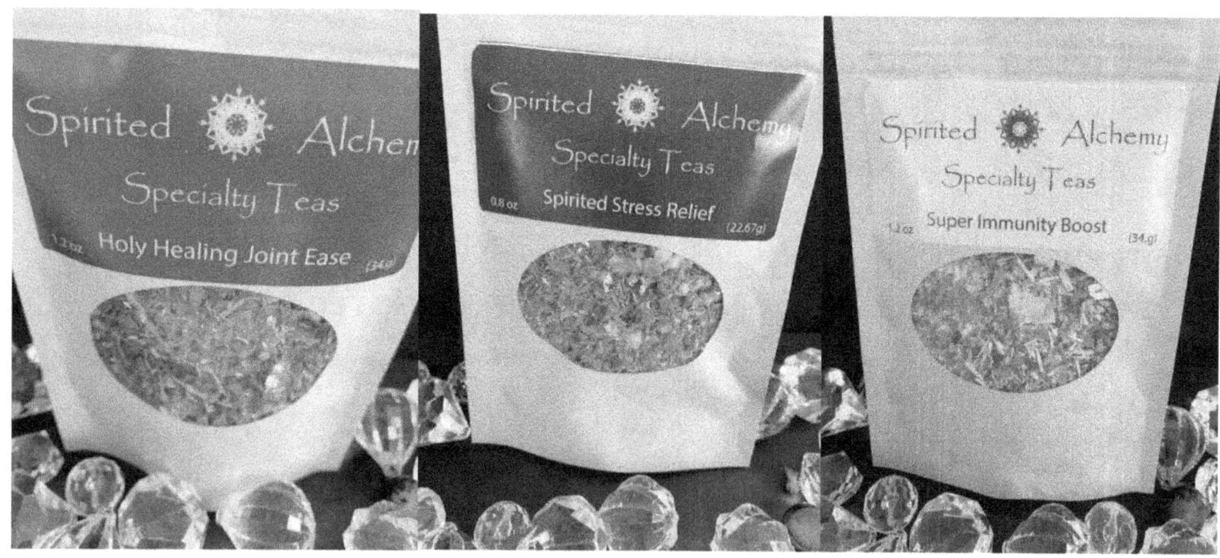

Holy Healing Joint Ease **Spirited Stress Relief** **Super Immunity Boost**

www.holyhealinghoney.com   www.holyhealingtea.com

Conclusion

Choosing the right herbal infusion that will suit your health needs and lifestyle can provide unlimited health benefits. You can drink to your health with a cup of herbal tea and know it's doing you good.

There are other herbal teas available also, some with similar properties to those listed, and some with different actions. Although there may be some herbal teas you may not like the taste of at first, the benefits that can be acquired from drinking herbal teas cannot be disputed.

In more books to come available on Spirited Alchemy of Tea I will have several ways to grow, plant, harvest and purchase your Herbs and Spices for Tea.

Obviously, each will have its own unique taste. It is also possible to blend your own teas, to combine different properties or tastes into the one cup.

To improve the taste, you can add some other healthy ingredients to fully enjoy your tea experience.

Experiment and create your very own super drink or order one of my health Spirited Alchemy Specialty Teas!

Best of Health

The Spirited Alchemy